PILATES
PLUS

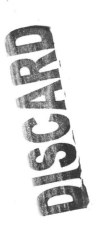

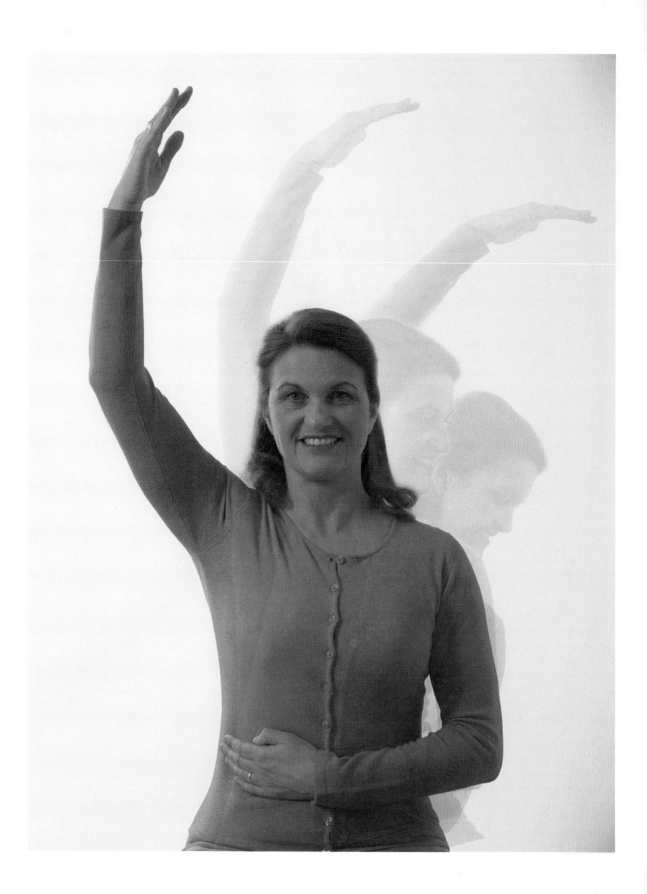

PILATES
PLUS

ALAN HERDMAN
with Gill Paul

Gaia Books

A GAIA ORIGINAL

Books from Gaia celebrate the vision of Gaia, the self-sustaining living Earth, and seek to help its readers live in greater personal and planetary harmony.

Editoral	**Susannah Steel**
Design	**Nick Harris**
Photography	**Paul Forrester**
Hair, make-up, and styling	**Richard Burns**
Production	**Louise Hall**
Picture Research	**Jennifer Veall**
Direction	**Jo Godfrey Wood, Patrick Nugent**

Registered trade mark of Gaia Books
An imprint of Octopus Publishing Group
2–4 Heron Quays, London, E14 4JP
Copyright © 2005 Gaia Books
Text copyright © 2005 Gaia Books
The right of Alan Herdman to be identified as the author of this work has been asserted in accordance with Sections 77 and 78 of the Copyright, Designs and Patents Act 1988, United Kingdom.
All rights reserved including the right of reproduction in whole or in part in any form.

First published in the United Kingdom by Gaia Books Ltd
Distributed in the United States and Canada by
Sterling Publishing Co., Inc.,
387 Park Avenue South, New York, NY 10016-8810
ISBN 1-85675-240-2
EAN 9 781856 752404
A catalogue record of this book is available from the British Library.
Printed and bound in Italy
10 9 8 7 6 5 4 3 2 1

Publisher's note The publisher and author specifically disclaim any responsibility for any liability, loss or risk which may be claimed or incurred as a consequence, directly or indirectly, of the use of any of the contents of this publication.

Contents

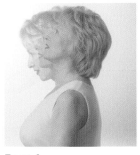
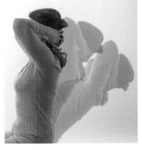
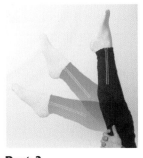
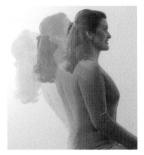

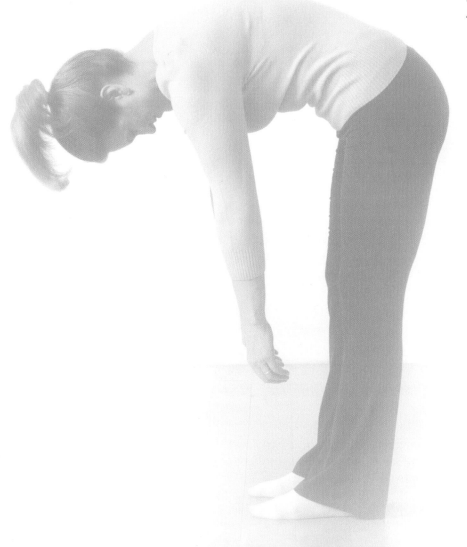

Introduction

According to Joseph Pilates, the founder of the Pilates exercise system, a person's true age is not measured in years, or how old they feel, but by the flexibility of their spine. If you are 30 years old and stiff as a plank of wood, with aching muscles and creaky joints, then you are elderly. If you are 70 years old, still leading an active life and able to twist and bend without aches and pains, then you are youthful.

Typically, our modern lifestyles don't tend to produce youthful 70 year olds. We rush to work, to the car, and then back home. We're preoccupied by watching television, doing housework and gardening, and talking on the telephone, not stopping to consider the physical side effects of all these activities until our bodies start to let us down. By the age of 20, the vast majority of people in the West have some degree of spinal curvature. This throws their entire body out of balance, although they probably won't feel the knock-on effects yet. However, at 50 most people will be aware of some physical weak spots. It might be a recurrent stiff neck in the morning, or "dodgy" knees, or nagging sciatica – or it could be something far more serious.

It goes to show just how resilient the human body is that bad postural habits can take years or even decades to become seriously debilitating. Even more amazing is that once habits are corrected, and the muscles are strengthened to hold the joints in correct alignment, you can reverse that damage in a matter of weeks. No matter what level of disability you suffer from, Pilates will create huge improvements if you are prepared to try. I can't emphasize enough that it is never too late to start Pilates; in fact, the more problems you have already, the faster you will begin to reap the benefits by doing this exercise.

Perhaps you have attempted to keep fit over the years by jogging in the park once a week, or by playing tennis, going to the gym, cycling, or exercising in front of keep-fit videos. If so, you may feel aggrieved when physical weaknesses set in. It doesn't seem fair! The problem is that these forms of exercise won't use all your muscles in a balanced way. They tend to focus on particular muscle groups – usually the larger ones – and they can become bulky and strong, to the detriment of the smaller muscles that are essential for overall flexibility. Trained athletes who try Pilates for the first time are astonished to find that they can hardly do any of the exercises properly. In Pilates, you learn to look after all your muscles, minor as well as major, and to balance the body. Your spine is held straight with the centre of gravity down the middle, not curving to one side or forwards or backwards.

Maybe you haven't exercised for years (or even decades). You've been too busy with your career or family, and could never find the time or inclination to join a gym. Perhaps you were put off by the sheer monotony of getting into a leotard or leggings and mindlessly pounding away until your muscles hurt. If this is the case, Pilates is the ideal way for you to regain muscle tone and fitness. It needn't take much time, you can do it when and where you like, it requires you to use your brain so you won't be bored, and it won't ever hurt if you perform the exercises correctly.

One of the greatest advantages of Pilates is that it will teach you self-sufficiency. All you need in order to do the various exercise sessions in this book is some loose, comfortable clothing to wear, a rug, yoga mat, or folded blanket to lie on, a few cushions and hand towels, a low stool, and a chair without arms. That's it! With this equipment, you can do Pilates exercises throughout the day, whenever you have a spare moment. You will also be taught to keep an awareness of your posture at all times.

This book will also enable you to treat your own aches and pains. If you wake up in the morning with lower back pain, you will be shown how to ease it out; if you suffer from arthritic hands, or osteoporosis, or painful feet, there is advice on exercises that can help to increase your range of movement.

Happily, Pilates is also good for the ego. Any flabby stomachs are firmed and flattened, and slouched shoulders are pulled back. Some people find that they even become taller as they straighten up their curved spines. All beginners see and feel a difference within the first few weeks – and that's a promise. It's a great rejuvenator. Isn't it time that you started turning back the clock?

The basic principles of Pilates

Joseph Pilates began developing his exercise system more than a hundred years ago to overcome some serious disabilities of his own: legs bowed by childhood rickets, a body stunted by rheumatic fever, and breathing difficulties caused by asthma. Pilates learned to cure himself first and then set about using what he had learned to help other people. During the First World War, he looked after injured patients in hospital and helped the bedridden regain mobility using ingenious devices made from bedsprings. In 1926, Pilates set up his first studio in New York, and taught his methods to a number of celebrity performers – including dancer Martha Graham and choreographer George Balanchine – to help their bodies withstand the rigours of their physically challenging profession. As the 20th century progressed and his reputation spread, he developed and adapted his techniques to deal with the range of problems that clients brought with them to his studio. Here are the basic components of Pilates' technique:

Concentration
You can't do Pilates exercises while thinking about anything else except your body. There are often several things to focus on at once, and you need to notice the way your muscles respond, and how it feels, to know if you are doing an exercise correctly.

Control
Pilates movements are all performed slowly and deliberately. There's no rushing to complete a set of repetitions in record time; it's much better to complete one perfect movement than ten haphazard ones. Some exercises look deceptively simple, but it can take weeks of practice to perform them perfectly.

Centre
Joseph Pilates called the muscles of the abdomen, hips, and buttocks the "powerhouse muscles". Many exercises are devoted to strengthening this area so that it can provide stability and support the body in everything that it is required to do.

Fluidity
Movements should never be jerky or erratic; they should always be as smooth and flowing as if you are dancing a waltz. During an exercise routine, even the links between different exercises should be performed gracefully and purposefully.

Precision

It is crucial that you always check and re-check the alignment of your body before starting an exercise. If you are only a couple of centimetres out of alignment, the movements will be much less effective. For optimum results, every single instruction in this book should be followed to the letter. And less is usually more: aim for small, clean movements rather than large, imprecise ones.

Breathing

Breathing fully and deeply will help to cleanse the lungs of stale air and get lots of fresh, energizing oxygen into the bloodstream. The Pilates method of breathing is designed to complement the exercises and make them even more effective.

Imagination

You need to be able to visualize the movements you want to make in order to perform them precisely. Once you can see a position in your mind's eye, it will be easier for you to find the muscles that will help you achieve it.

Intuition

As you learn Pilates, you will learn more about your body – its strengths, weaknesses, asymmetries, and capabilities. So, when a movement feels difficult or you get a twinge in a joint, you will understand how to self-diagnose and take action to fix it yourself. Awareness of your body will also help you to judge when a problem requires medical advice.

Integration

Although you will learn to isolate a particular muscle group, you should always be thinking about the body as a whole. When working on your thighs, for example, you should be aware of the position of your arms; while stretching your neck, you should feel the weight of your body evenly balanced in your feet. This is easier than it sounds if you work slowly and smoothly, integrating breathing with all the movements that you are instructed to make.

Don't feel as though you have to memorize all these principles before you go any further. So long as you have a general awareness of what Pilates is about, and you don't approach it like yet another aerobics or step class, you won't go wrong. If you haven't tried it before, open your mind and realize that it's going to be different from any exercise system you've ever come across before – and get ready to experience some dramatic results.

About the author

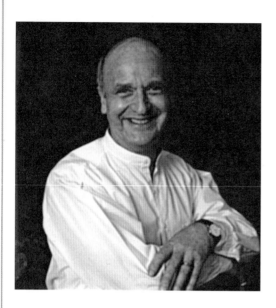

I learned the Pilates method from two of Joseph Pilates' protégés, Bob Fitzgerald and Carola Trier, just after Joseph Pilates died in 1967, and I brought it across the Atlantic to open the UK's first Pilates studio in 1970. Since then, I have continued to adapt and develop new exercises to address the needs of every client I consult with. (You can read some of their stories on pages 132–35.) I have worked with actors, dancers, musicians, doctors, dentists, journalists, builders, and sportsmen and women – all kinds of people with a huge variety of physical problems. I use a piece of equipment called a "reformer" in my studio – a kind of supportive exercise machine with springs, based on the prototypes Pilates developed – but I always train each client in mat work first. This means that they have an understanding of all the correct techniques required to be able to do Pilates at home. Sometimes new problems call for new solutions, but the principles that Joseph Pilates established in the early 20th century remain the core of my work.

How to use this book

If you are over 40 years old and haven't exercised for some time, or if you have a pre-existing health condition for which you are receiving medical treatment, consult your doctor or specialist before starting any new exercise regime. Part 3 of this book deals with some specific physical problems, and gives advice on movements you should emphasize, and those you should avoid, both during exercise sessions and in daily life. If you know that you have a joint weakness, a tendency to back pain, or a health condition, read the appropriate section in part 3 before trying any of the exercises in the rest of the book.

If you don't have any specific complaints, you can begin with part 1 and work your way through the book, carefully trying each movement as you go. All the models in this book are 50 years old or more, so be encouraged to try all the exercises. It may help to keep a notebook so that you can list those exercises you find tricky, as well as the ones you can manage easily, so that you can identify areas that require more work. Be honest about your capabilities. You're not trying to break any world records, and you won't achieve results any faster by racing through the exercises. You need to truly understand what you're doing, and why. We're not giving out medals, and it doesn't matter if your friend or partner looks more proficient than you. This is simply about making your body as supple and as strong as it can possibly be.

Start to integrate the correct posture, as explained in part 1, into your daily life, and go through the Top-to-toe workout in part 2 very slowly. As you do each exercise, stop to make sure that you can feel the right muscles working. This is so that you can create a "memory" of the sensations for future reference. Once you have mastered each of the Top-to-toe exercises (this may take a few weeks for beginners), try the workouts in part 4. You can also develop your own exercises to fit the time you have available and how you're feeling on the day. Always exercise on a carpet or a non-slip surface, using a yoga mat if necessary.

Pilates has a side effect that we haven't discussed so far, and that is the way in which it makes you feel calmer, less stressed, and more in control of your own well-being. Rather than try to explain this aspect further, I'm going to let you start the learning process instead and find out for yourselves. Get ready to change your life.

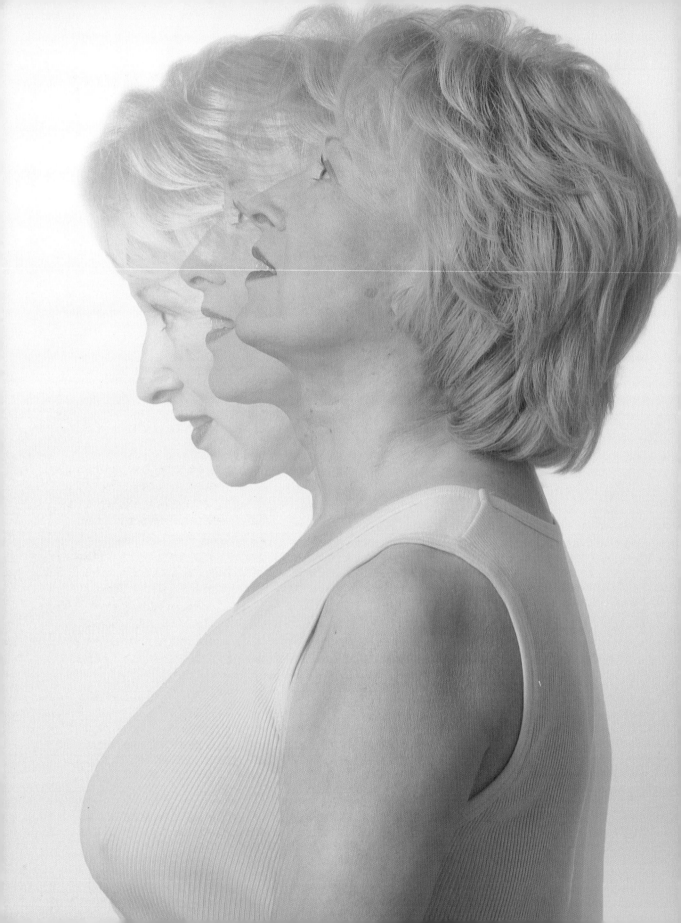

PART **1**

The Pilates lifestyle

In almost every activity we undertake in life, we have a tendency to misuse our bodies. Spending time working on computers, driving long distances in the car, doing housework, shopping in super-markets — even brushing your teeth and washing your face in the morning — can strain your back. The purpose of this chapter is to show you the Pilates way of doing common, everyday tasks safely and comfortably, without causing joint imbalance and muscle strain. For a few weeks you might have to think through each movement first, but before long it should become second nature to you.

To start with, you will need to diagnose any existing postural imperfections. Almost everyone has some, including top athletes, dancers, gymnasts and the majority of people in their twenties. These postural imperfections will affect the way you sit, stand, move, and breathe. If you believe that you have perfect posture, you could be in for a few surprises because most of us are far less symmetrical than we think.

13

Assessing your posture

Put on a t-shirt and some leggings, or any other outfit that enables you to see your shape clearly. Stand up straight in front of a full-length mirror. It may help if you can do this with a partner or a friend who will intervene when you are feeling less than objective about yourself.
Answer these questions:

Is one shoulder higher than the other?

If so, hunch your shoulders up to your ears and let them slide down slowly. Are they the same height now? If not, you could have tightness on one side of your neck and shoulders, or an imbalance in the muscles of your back.

When your arms hang loosely at your sides, are the fingers of each hand at the same level?

If not, this could be another sign that you're holding one shoulder higher than the other, and you need to focus on shoulder release, neck and upper back exercises (see pp.82–86).

Are your hip bones level, or are you leaning slightly to one side?

One way to check this is to see whether the gap between your wrists and your hips is the same on both sides. There can be several reasons why you might lean more of your weight onto one hip: it could mean you have scoliosis, or uneven leg lengths, or it could just be that years of poor postural habits have caused the muscles to shorten on one side. You will need to strengthen the muscles of the stomach and pelvic area to help you balance your weight more evenly (see pp.90–93).

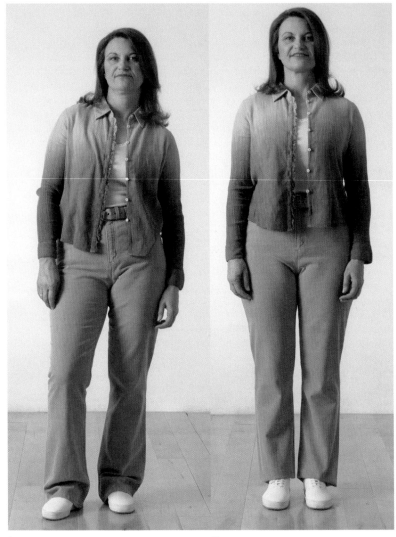

Incorrect posture

Correct posture

Are your kneecaps facing forward or are they rotated outward or inward?

You're at risk of knee injuries if the knees are rotated, and you'll be knocking your hips out of alignment as well; but strengthening the leg muscles will help you to correct this problem (see pp.96–100).

Are you balancing your weight squarely across your feet, or are you rolling your weight inward, outward, forward, or backward?

Feet problems affect the knees, hips, and spine, and have knock-on effects throughout the body. See pages 102–103 for more ways to test whether your weight is correctly balanced through your feet.
Now stand sideways to the mirror.

14

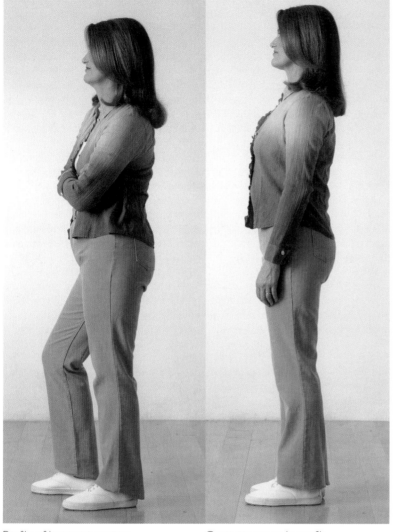

Profile of incorrect posture   Correct posture in profile

Before starting any Pilates exercise, you should stop and mentally check your posture and alignment. It's a good idea to do this throughout the day whenever you remember. Visualize the shape of your spine right now. Is it twisted to one side, arched, or hunched over? Imagine a piece of string going straight up the centre of your spine, emerging through the crown of your head. Think of pulling that string straight and taut, and your posture will improve instantly.

Does your chin jut outward or upward?

It should be level and pulled back slightly so that your spine is straight and your head is slightly forward from the top of the spine. If it's not, you may need to focus on neck, shoulder, and upper back exercises to correct your posture (see pp.82–86).

Do your shoulders and/or your upper back seem to curl forward?

This can indicate a condition called kyphosis, about which there is advice on page 82.

Look at the curve of your spine at waist level. Is it pronounced, causing your bottom to stick out? Is your stomach hanging out or is it reasonably flat?

Pronounced curves in the lower spine can indicate a condition called lordosis (see p.89).

Sitting in chairs

A well-designed chair is the first requirement for achieving a safe, comfortable sitting posture. Huge sofas that are low in height and covered with cushions may look tempting, but it's almost impossible to sit in them without slumping into your lower back or twisting and crossing your legs. Look instead for a chair that is the same height as the lower half of your legs (from knee to heel), and with a seat that is the length of your thighs. Go to a showroom and test a few for comfort. Look for "medium firm": not too hard and not too soft.

When you sit on a chair, your back should be positioned right at the back of the chair, with your feet resting firmly on the ground. If there is a space between your back and the chair back, insert a cushion. Rest the backs of your thighs on the chair so that your weight is transmitted through them and down to your feet. Your hip and knee joints should be bent at right angles.

CAUTION: After a hip replacement operation, you will need a high seat so that you can sit with your hips higher than your knees.

Sitting down

Safely sitting down on a chair is all about weight distribution.

1 Stand in front of the chair with your feet flat on the floor and hip-width apart. Keep your back straight.

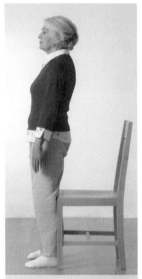

2 Draw your stomach muscles in and bend forward from the waist while aiming your bottom back toward the seat. You can lean on the arm rests or place your hands on your thighs, but get that feeling of leaning forward, then leading the way with your bottom. Keep your back straight; don't let it curve forward.

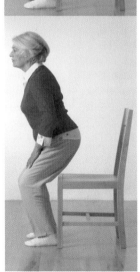

Standing up

Several muscle groups are involved in the process of standing up from a sitting position.

1 Make sure that your feet are flat on the floor, and about hip-width apart. Engage your stomach muscles and lean forward from the waist, keeping a straight spine.

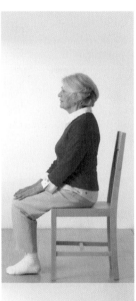

2 Once your weight is well forward, use your stomach muscles, glutes, and thigh muscles to pitch your weight off your thighs and onto your feet. You can push on the arm rests if you like, or place your hands on your thighs. Push down with your hands as you lift upward.

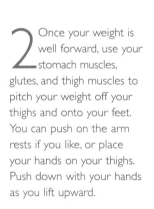
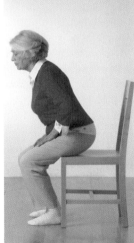

Working at a desk

Some people spend around 40 hours a week sitting at a desk reading, writing, talking on the phone, or working at a computer. Bad postural habits while working could quickly undo the benefits of a couple of hours of Pilates exercises a week, so whether you have any problems yet or not, it makes sense to think about the way you spend your working life.

Make sure that your chair is the right height for your feet to rest flat on the floor, your back to rest against the chair back, and your knees and hips to be at right angles. Your forearms should be able to rest on your desk when you bend your elbows 90 degrees. Make sure your chair is near enough to the desk so that you don't reach forward to work.

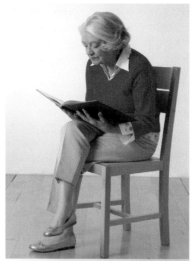

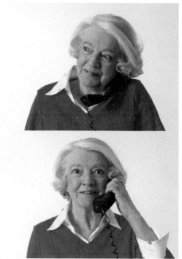

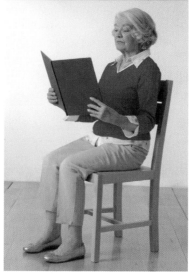

Using the telephone

If you spend a lot of time using the phone, you should invest in a hands-free set (or ask your boss to do so). Holding a handset to one ear regularly is going to create a muscle imbalance, unless you are careful to keep your shoulders and wrists relaxed and your neck and back straight. Whatever you do, don't cradle the phone between your ear and your shoulder to free up your hands. If you could see all the structures you are crushing inside your neck, you would never do this again.

Using a computer

Position the screen directly in front of you. The centre of the screen should be at eye level so that you don't have to look up, down, or sideways. Keep the keyboard straight in front of you so that when you type you keep your elbows by your sides and your wrists straight. The mouse should be within easy reach, and there should be space to rest your forearms on the desk.

Reading and writing

Instead of bending your neck to look at your paperwork, invest in a tilted drawing board so you can arrange your papers at eye level, and hold them in place with a clip or a magnet. This is important if you suffer from osteoporosis or kyphosis, but it's good practice for anyone. How are you holding this book? When reading, hold the book at eye level instead of resting it on a desk or on your lap. If this strains your neck, shoulders, or arms, buy an upright book rest.

Don't work in the same position for longer that 20–30 minutes without a break. From time to time, refocus your eyes by looking out of a window, at a picture on the wall, or at a colleague. Get up and walk around, or do a few loosening-up exercises at your desk. Shrug your shoulders to your ears. Pull your stomach muscles toward the back of the chair. Squeeze your glutes. Do the Cossack Arms exercise (see p.33), or Sitting lats exercises (see p.63). Once you are familiar with Pilates, you will be able to choose your own exercises to relieve stiffness.

Flexibility

If you maintain flexibility in your spine, you'll look and feel much younger than contemporaries of yours who haven't done so. There's nothing quite so ageing as moaning and clutching your back as you bend to pick something up from the carpet, or try to put on your socks in the morning.

Try this spine roll-down exercise and note any points at which you feel stiffness. Stop altogether if you feel any sharp pain, and only go as far as you can manage comfortably. You can rest against a wall or door as you do this exercise if you're worried about over-balancing.

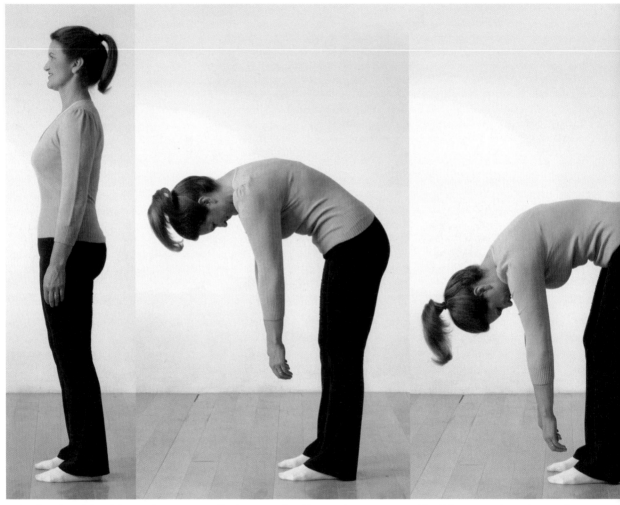

1 Stand straight with your feet apart, approximately in line with your hip joints. Keep your knees "soft" (that is, slightly bent). Hold your stomach in and let your chin roll down to your chest.

2 Let your shoulders and arms hang forwards in front of you. Then slowly let your upper back drop down toward the floor, gradually stretching your spine and keeping your knees slightly bent.

3 When your fingertips touch the floor, or as far as you can manage, stop, breathe in, then pull your stomach muscles in again. Tuck your bottom under to begin rolling back up again, straightening your spine section by section.

Balance

CAUTION: Don't try this exercise if you suffer from osteoporosis.

Your weight may appear to be evenly balanced across your hips when you're standing still, but this might not be the case when you're walking. The muscles might be weaker on one side than the other. Try this exercise to find out how good your balance is. If you discover one side is weaker, make a note that it will need extra work. It's important to keep the posture muscles strong.

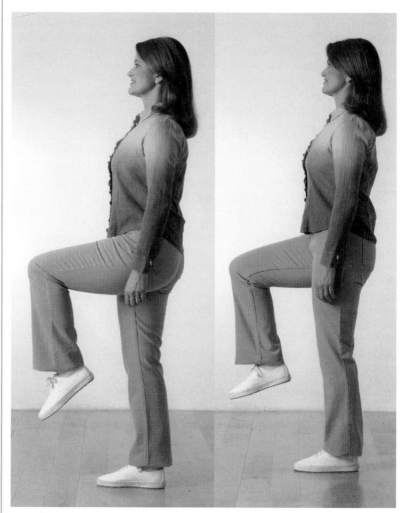

4 As you return to an upright position, let your shoulders slide back and lengthen your neck.

1 Stand up straight with your arms by your sides, hip bones level and feet hip-width apart. Pull your stomach muscles in. Lift your left leg off the floor and balance your weight evenly through your right foot, without sinking into your right hip. Try to keep your hip bones level. Hold for a few seconds. Are you wobbling? Put your left leg down again.

2 Now lift your right leg off the floor and balance your weight through the left foot. Are you more stable on your right leg, or less stable, or are they about the same? When you do leg exercises, include more repetitions on the weaker side.

Breathing

Picture your lungs as a couple of pink balloons inside your chest. If you breathe in deeply, with your shoulders relaxed and head held straight, the balloons can inflate fully and allow the maximum amount of oxygen into your bloodstream. As you breathe out, you should deflate the balloons completely and expel all the waste carbon dioxide from your system. So far, so good.

On the other hand, if you take quick, shallow breaths with the shoulders hunched forward and your chin jutting upwards, you'll only manage to inflate the balloons slightly. There'll be a bit of air in them at the top, but they won't be able to pass much oxygen to all the blood vessels that supply the muscles, heart, brain, and other organs.

Good posture is essential for your lungs to work efficiently. As you breathe in, your ribs should expand outward and backward; then, as you breathe out, they should come inward and forward. Keeping your spine straight will prevent your shoulders hunching and your ribs collapsing into your stomach as you breathe out.

Here are two ways to test how effectively you are breathing.

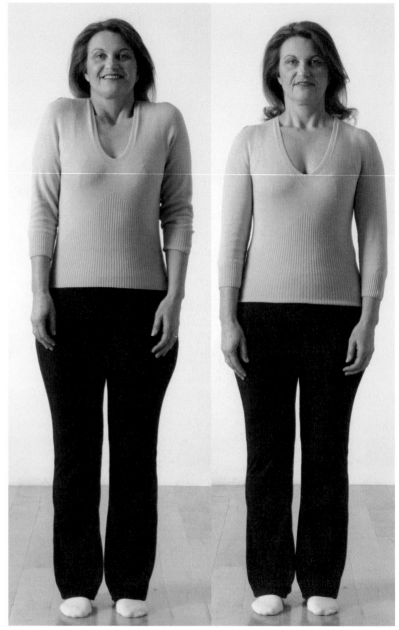

Stand up straight in front of a mirror with relaxed shoulders. Hunch them up to your ears and let them slide down if you need to relax them. Take a full breath in through your nose and watch your shoulders. Do they rise up as you breathe in? They should stay completely still while your ribs make the movements. Breathe in again through your nose and look at your neck. Are there any signs of strain, such as tendons standing out? This could be the case if your breathing muscles are weak.

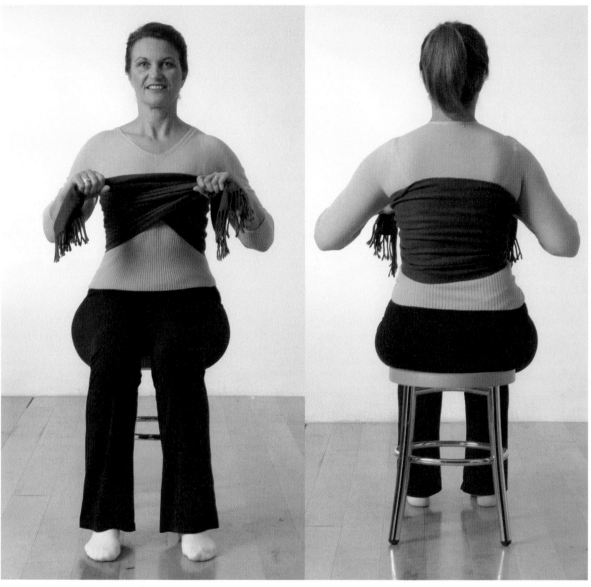

2 You will need a scarf and a firm, armless chair or stool for this test. Sit upright with feet apart. Position the scarf around your upper back so that it covers the area just underneath the arms down to the base of the ribs. Cross over the ends of the scarf and hold them firmly in each hand. Breathe in through your nose and try to feel your ribs pushing against the scarf. Now breathe out through your mouth in a slow, controlled manner and feel your ribs move back in again as you tighten the scarf around you.

Keep practising this scarf breathing to ensure that you are using the correct breathing muscles. There are more breathing exercises on pages 87–88. During Pilates exercises, you will usually be asked to breathe in through your nose during the preparation for a movement, then out through your mouth as you perform the movement.

Finding your abdominals

Most Pilates exercises require you to hold your stomach muscles in before you perform the movement, thus protecting your spine. However, if your stomach is flabby and the muscles weak, you may find it difficult to do this effectively. Some people who come to my studio can't even find their stomach muscles at first, but they're always amazed how quickly they can control them if they practise regularly.

Give it a try right now, while sitting reading this book. Place your hands loosely on your thighs, make sure your spine is straight, then breathe out and pull your stomach towards the back of the chair. Can you pull it in so that it is flat, or even slightly concave? You can do this basic exercise anywhere: while standing in a queue at the bank, driving, or sitting at your desk. One of the great things about the focus Pilates puts on strong stomach muscles is that everyone who practises diligently will see a difference within three weeks of starting. Don't set impossible goals; if you've got a naturally curvaceous figure, your stomach may always be slightly rounded, but it should be firm rather than wobbly.

Did you have trouble pulling your stomach muscles toward the back of the chair? If so, you should find them easier to control in this next exercise that I want you to try.

Side-lying static abs

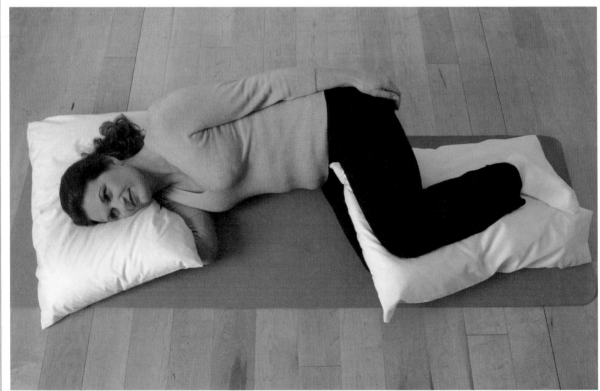

1 Lie on one side with your knees bent, and your feet in line with your tailbone. Place a pillow between your head and your lower arm, and another between your thighs.

2 Relax your stomach so that it flops down toward the floor. Let it all hang out! Breathe in.

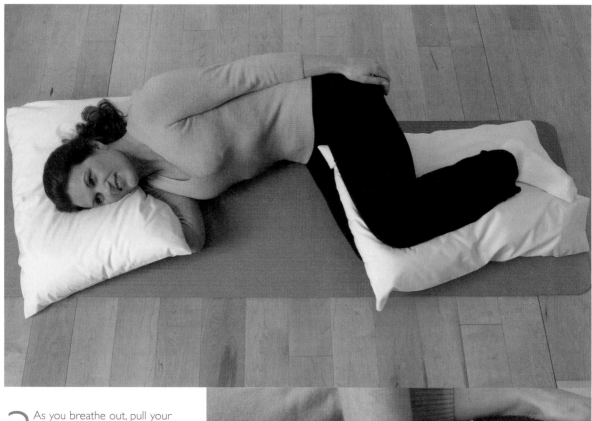

3 As you breathe out, pull your stomach up, away from the floor and back toward your spine in a kind of L-shaped movement. Repeat this exercise 10 times.

4 By pulling in your stomach – as if you have an instructor's hand pulling your muscles back into shape – you pull the oblique and transverse muscles of your abdominal region up and in.

Turn onto your other side, rearrange the pillows, check your position, and do 10 repetitions.

When you are told in an exercise to "engage" your stomach muscles, it will refer to this action of pulling your stomach towards your back. Practise pulling your stomach muscles in whenever you have a spare moment.

Finding your glutes

The gluteus maximus muscles (we'll call them glutes), which extend across your buttocks, are crucial for walking and keeping your pelvis in the correct position. Older people can be prone to tripping over if their glutes aren't strong because they have to tilt their pelvis in order to lift each leg off the ground.

Find your glutes right now by squeezing your buttocks together. Can you squeeze the muscles strongly enough to feel as though they are gently touching each other? Here are a couple of exercises to help you strengthen them – and, as a welcome side effect, they can make your bottom look more pert.

Standing glute squeeze

1 Rest your hands against a wall or on the back of a chair, or hold onto a doorway for support. Your feet should be parallel and roughly hip-width apart. Breathe out and squeeze your buttocks together. Hold the squeeze for four seconds. You will feel a pull on the inner thigh muscles, but don't let your legs rotate outward.

2 Breathe in, then repeat. Feel the way your pelvis adjusts slightly and your stomach muscles automatically engage. Repeat 10 times.

If one side feels weaker than the other, squeeze the weak side first and then the stronger one. They should even up in time.

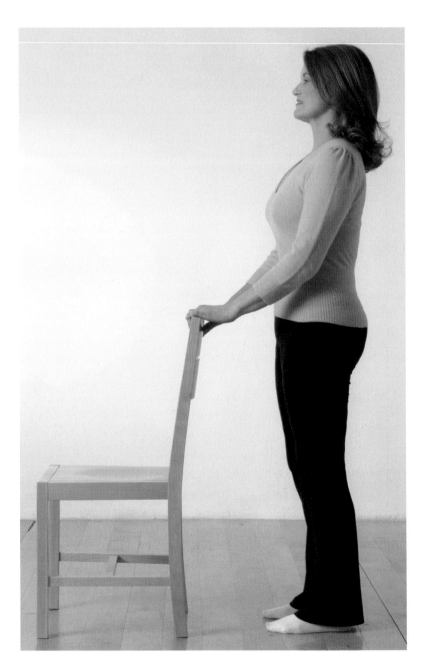

The Bridge

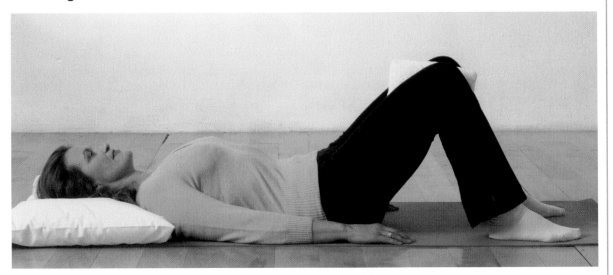

1   Lie on your back on the floor with your knees bent. Your feet should be flat and roughly hip-width apart. Place a small folded towel between your thighs to keep this width consistent. Rest your head on a pillow or folded towel so that your neck is straight. Relax your arms by your sides and let your shoulders sink into the floor. Breathe in.

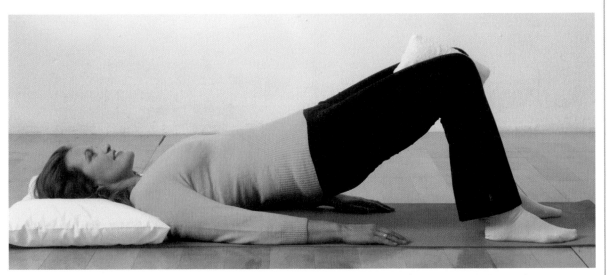

2   As you breathe out, engage your stomach muscles, gently lift your pelvis a few centimetres off the floor, and squeeze your glutes. Hold for four seconds, then release gently. If you feel this movement pulling in your lower back, don't lift so high – or avoid this exercise until your stomach muscles are stronger.

Now that you have found how to isolate and engage two of the most important muscle groups for "core stability", we're going to look at the ways in which they can help you to perform everyday activities efficiently, without straining.

Are you sleeping comfortably?

Restful sleep is essential for good health, and you will only sleep well if you are comfortable in your bed. Ensure that your mattress is "medium firm", that is, neither too hard, which would force the bones into odd alignments, nor too soft, so you sink into dips and hollows. If you roll into the middle of the bed every night, your mattress is too soft. Mattresses should be turned every few months and replaced at least every ten years so that you avoid a saggy bed.

If you ever get back pain – even just a niggle – then the best sleeping position for taking a nap or sleeping during the night is lying on your side with your knees bent in a loose foetal position. Place a pillow of the right thickness under your head so that you keep your spine in a straight line. If you place a pillow between your legs, the pelvis will be held in the correct position as you sleep, and won't pull on your lower back. Alternatively, if you like to lie on your side with the top leg bent over and the lower leg straight, place a pillow under the knee of the top leg.

Lower back stretch

When you wake in the morning or from a nap, try to make time for a few simple stretches to loosen up your muscles. You'll need to take only five minutes to do them, and you will definitely feel the difference. If you do this sequence in bed, push the covers aside first.

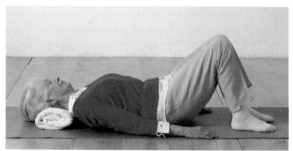

1 Lie on your back with your knees bent. Place a folded towel under your head. Relax your arms on the floor and breathe in.

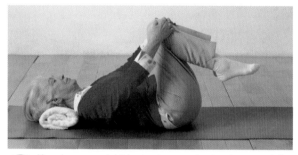

3 Keeping your right knee at your chest, raise your left knee as well and hold your knees so that they are parallel, but slightly apart. Breathe in.

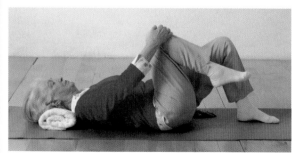

2 As you breathe out, engage your abdominals and lift the right knee up toward your chest. Hold it with your right hand, feeling the stretch in your lower back. Your right thigh should be at right angles to the floor.

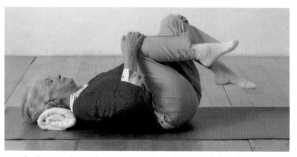

4 As you breathe out, gently pull your right knee towards your chest. Breathe in to relax, then release your right knee a little.

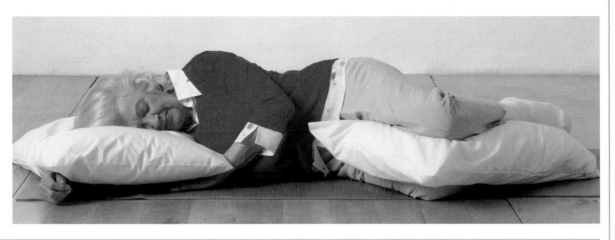

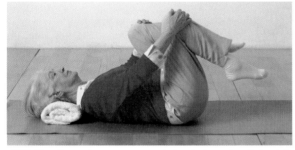

5 Breathe out, engage your abdominals, and pull the left knee toward your chest. Breathe in to relax, then release the left knee a little.

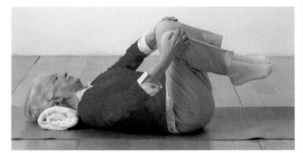

7 Press your knees together and imagine that your lower back is resting on a clock face. Slowly circle your knees four times in a clockwise direction, then circle them another four times anticlockwise. Breathe easily throughout this movement.

Lower your right leg to the floor first, then let your left leg follow. Don't ever lower them both at the same time.

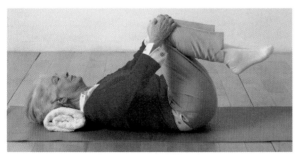

6 Now breathe out and pull both knees together toward your chest.

Circulation stimulators

Leaping out of bed to the sound of the alarm clock can make you feel dizzy, as your circulation struggles to cope with the switch from horizontal to vertical. This can be pronounced for anyone with poor circulation or a heart condition. Try the following movements to stretch your muscles and give your blood a chance to reach the extremities before you get out of bed.

Back release

1 As you lie on the bed, kick off the covers. Breathe out, engage your abdominals, and bend your left knee. Stretch your left arm back behind you. Breathe in and, as you breathe out, slide your foot until your leg is fully extended again.

2 Breathe out, engage your abdominals, bend your right knee and stretch out your right arm. Breathe out and extend your leg.

Repeat three times on each side.

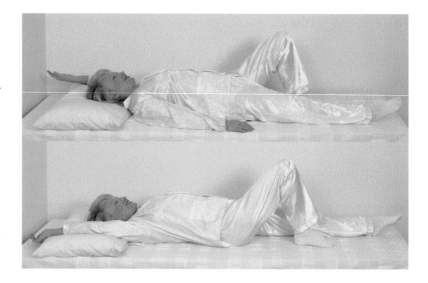

Lower back stretch

1 Lie on your back with your arms at your sides and breathe in. As you breathe out, engage your abdominals and lift one knee toward your chest, then the other. Place your hands on your knees. Breathe in. Breathe out and draw the right knee further toward your chest. Breathe in, then release so that your knees are aligned.

2 Breathe out and draw the left knee further toward your chest. Breathe in, then release to align your knees once more. Breathe out and bring both knees in toward your chest. Breathe in, then release and rest both feet on the bed.

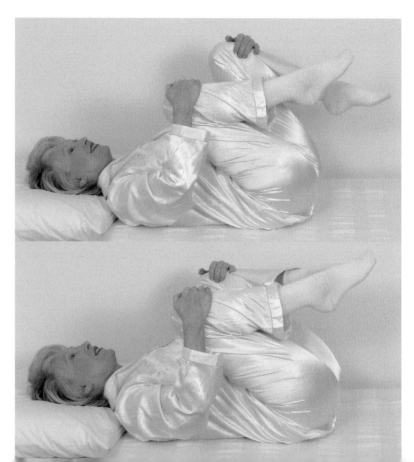

Hip rolls

1 Lie on your back with your arms at your sides. Bend your knees and keep your feet flat on the bed.

2 Breathe out, engage your abdominals, and let your legs drop gently down to the right. Keep your torso still and breathe in. Breathe out as you return to the start position.

Repeat three times on each side.

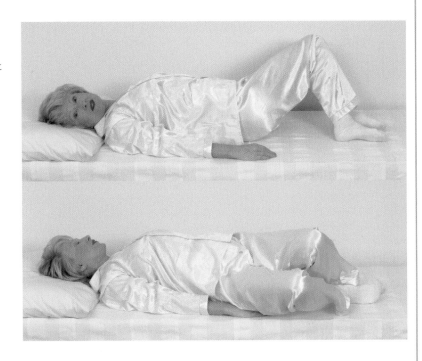

Point and flex

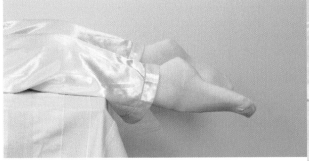

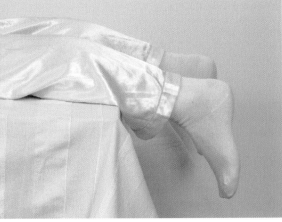

1 Turn over onto your stomach and wriggle down the bed so that your feet are hanging off the end, or swivel round so that they extend over the side. If necessary, place a pillow under your stomach to support your lower back. Point the toes of both feet and hold for a few seconds, but don't strain so hard that you get cramp. Gently does it.

CAUTION: If you find it difficult to lie on your stomach, do the Point and flex exercise lying on your back with one pillow supporting your head and another beneath your knees.

2 Flex the toes back, feeling the pull in your calf muscles. Hold for a few seconds. Repeat two or three times.

Circle the left ankle three times in a clockwise direction, then three times anticlockwise. Repeat with the right ankle.

Getting out of bed

If you have any kind of joint problem, or you are prone to stiffness, follow these steps carefully when getting out of bed.

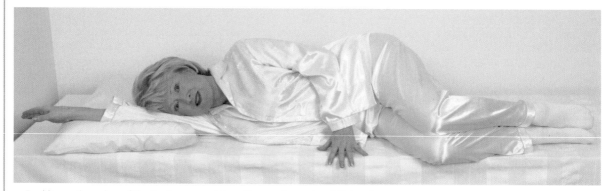

1 Lie on the edge of the bed on one side, with your knees bent. Extend your lower arm along the bed with the palm facing down and rest your head on your arm. Hold the edge of the bed with your free hand. Slide your lower legs outward, then down toward the floor, still keeping your head on the pillow.

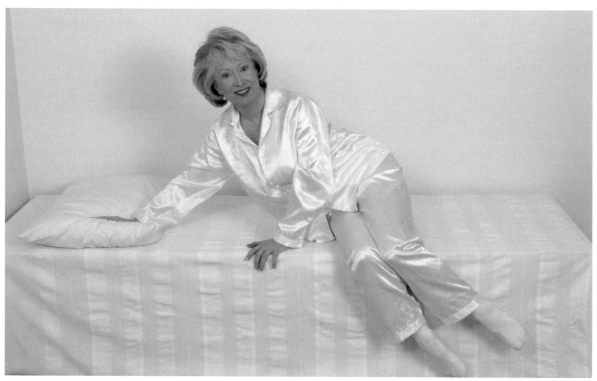

2 Use your arms to gradually push your torso into an upright position as you slowly lower your legs down to the ground.

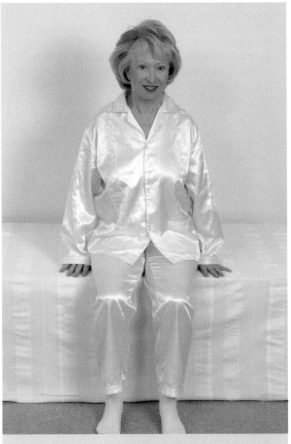

3 Continue to use your arms to push yourself up until you are in a sitting position with your feet firmly on the floor.

4 Shrug your shoulders up to your ears and let them slide down gently. Repeat a few times. This is a good precursor to many Pilates exercises, helping you to relax your shoulders, but you should also do it at any point during the day when you feel a bit stiff, or have been in the same position for a while.

Don't stand up yet – on the next page there are some stretches you can do to loosen up while sitting on the edge of the bed.

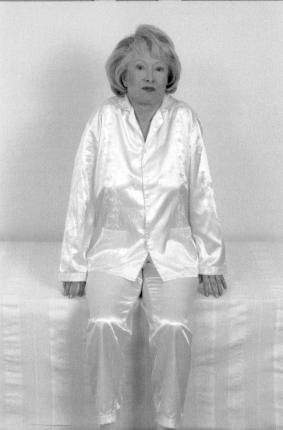

Edge of the bed stretches

You can either sit on the edge of the bed or on a low chair or stool for these gentle but effective stretches. Wherever you sit, keep your feet flat on the floor throughout.

Neck stretch

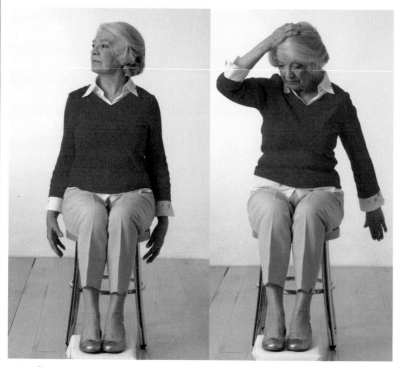

Thoracic stretch

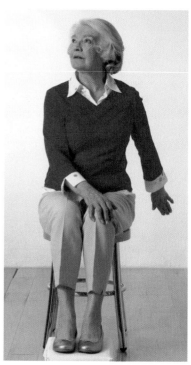

1   Sit up straight so that your thighs are parallel to the floor. If necessary, place a book or yoga block under your feet. Let your arms hang by your sides. Turn your head slightly to the right.

CAUTION: If you are being treated for a neck problem, check with your doctor or physio before doing any neck stretches.

2   Place your right hand on top of your head. Pull your head slightly further to the right until you feel a stretch in the tendons down the left side of your neck. Keep your nose in line with your right elbow.

Repeat on the other side, turning your head to the left, and placing your left hand over the top of your head.

1   Bring your right hand across the body to rest on your left knee. Let your left arm hang down toward the floor. Rotate it backward and you will feel a gentle stretch in your back.

Cossack Arms

1 Sit up straight with your elbows out at the sides and your palms facing downward. Touch your fingertips together in front of your breastbone. Think of pulling your shoulder blades down your back and relaxing your shoulders and neck completely. Breathe in.

2 As you breathe out, engage your abdominals and slowly turn your upper body round to the right. Keep your fingertips in front of your breastbone and your spine straight. Don't try to turn too far, and keep your knees still. If your arms become heavy, rest your hands on your thighs and continue.

Breathe in and return to the starting position. Repeat in the other direction.

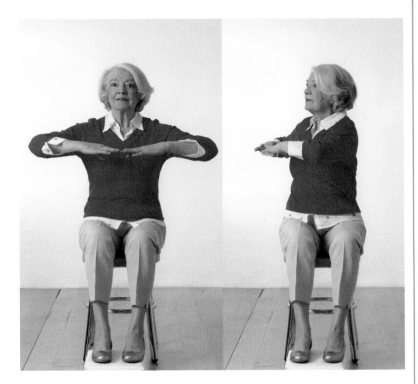

Side stretch

1 Sit up straight with your feet firmly on the floor about hip-width apart. Place your right hand on your ribs, just under the armpit. Curve your left arm above your head and look slightly to the right. Alternatively, you can bend your arm and rest your hand on your head if you find this easier. Breathe in.

2 As you breathe out, engage your stomach muscles and stretch to the right so that your left elbow rises towards the ceiling. Don't try to go too far – just stretch until you can feel the ribs opening up on your left side.

Breathe in and return to the starting position. Repeat, stretching to the left.

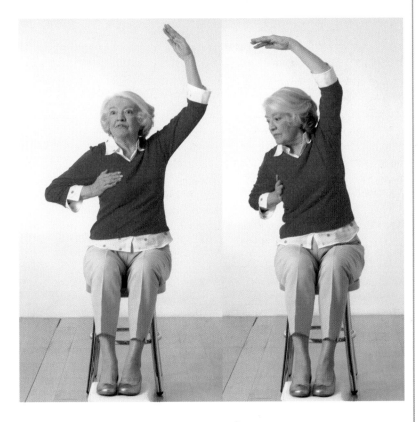

At the wash basin

It's easy to hunch your shoulders and curve your upper spine forward as you perform your morning toilette, thus forcing your upper back into a pronounced curve and making your bottom stick out. This position would be bad news for anyone, but particularly so if you have existing upper or lower back problems, or you suffer from osteoporosis.

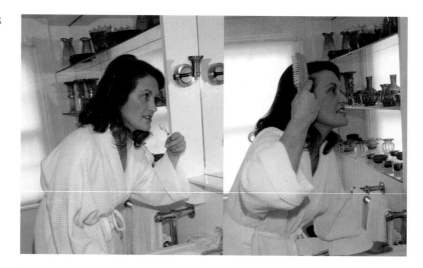

Upstairs, downstairs

From a postural point of view, most people don't climb stairs well. They hang onto a hand rail, lean their weight forward, and let their legs do all the work. It is much kinder to the body if you use your stomach muscles, glutes, and leg muscles together as you climb.

1 Hold your stomach in, make sure your back is straight, and slightly squeeze your glutes as you lift one leg onto the first step. Don't lean forwards – try to stay vertical. As you lift, balance your weight down into the back leg for a second or two. You should try to do this while keeping your pelvis level, as in the balance test on page 19.

2 Transfer your weight to the higher leg as you lift your lower leg, still keeping your back upright. Use a hand rail if you wish, but don't lean your weight into it.

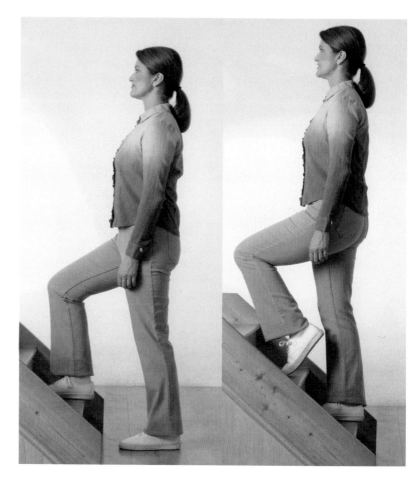

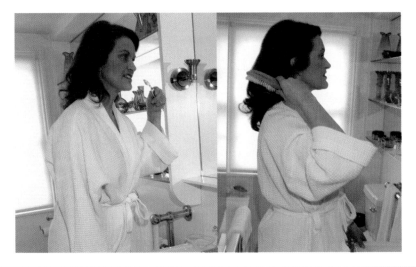

A better way of leaning over a basin to wash your face or brush your teeth is to stand with one leg in front of the other. Bend forward from the waist, keeping your spine straight. Hold onto the basin with one hand if you need to, and hold your stomach in to help maintain good posture.

When brushing your hair, avoid leaning your head to one side to resist the pull of the brush. Keep your back straight and your shoulders relaxed.

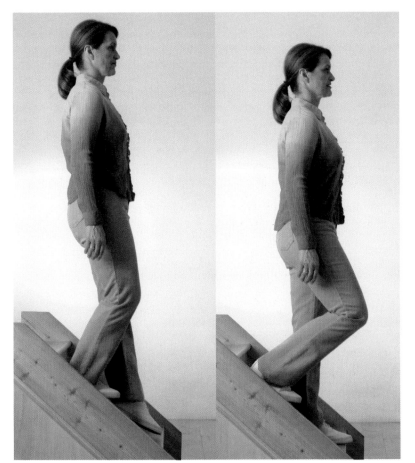

Going downstairs, the procedure is similar:

1 Point your toes and stretch one leg to the step below, simultaneously bending your other leg and using your stomach muscles to support you.

2 Place your foot flat on the step. Lift and bend the other leg, transferring your weight onto your flat foot.

CAUTION: If you have a weakness in one leg or hip, always lead with the good leg when going upstairs and with the bad leg when going down. The simple rule is that the bad leg should be on the lower step. As you become stronger, you can try letting the weaker leg do the work for a few steps at a time.

Lifting and carrying

If, for any peculiar reason, you wanted to put your back out, one of the easiest ways would be to try to lift a heavy box by leaning over it with straight legs and a rounded back. If you were twisting at an angle to reach it, you would be even more likely to cause damage. Follow these steps to lift and carry properly.

To lift a heavy object

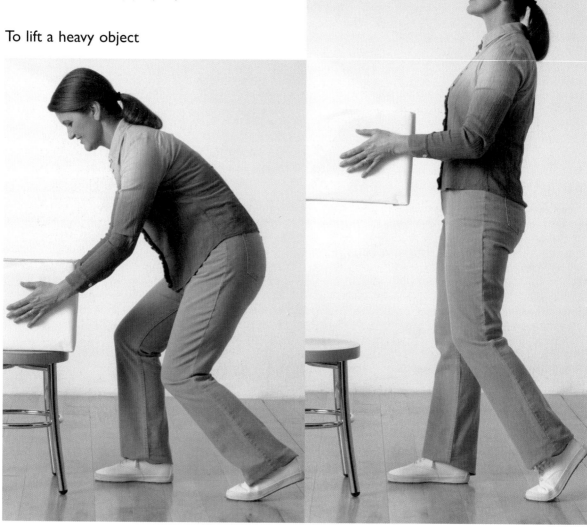

Make sure that the object is directly in front of you and as close to you as possible. Position your feet hip-width apart and step forward with one foot. Bend your knees until you are at the same level as the object, keeping your front foot flat on the floor. Hold the object with both hands. Let your legs do the work of lifting you back up while you concentrate on keeping your back straight.

To carry heavy bags

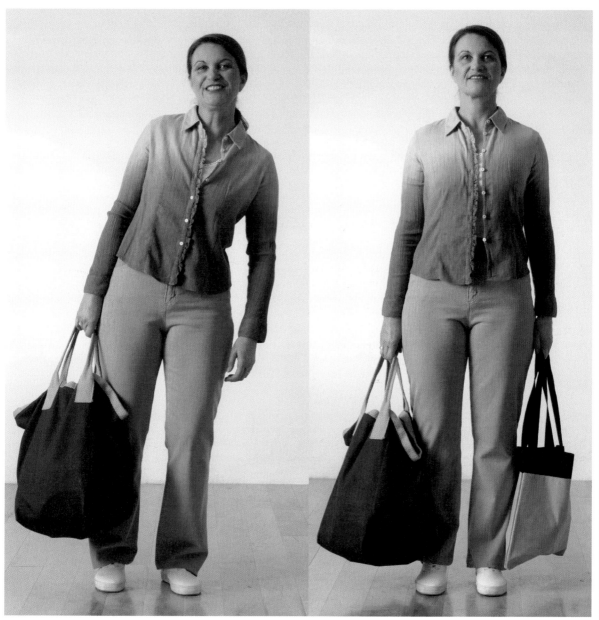

Try to avoid this situation, if at all possible. If you have no choice, spread the load between two bags and hold one bag in each hand for balance. Keep your elbows slightly bent rather than locked, so that you don't strain the joints. Never use a bag that hangs from one shoulder – the knock-on effects on your neck, spine, and pelvis are not pleasant. A small knapsack worn on your back and secured over both shoulders will spread the load more easily.

Lifting and carrying

It's all too easy to hunch your shoulders and lock your knees as you bend over the washing machine, or take a dish or casserole out of a low oven. Straight legs and a crunched neck are no way to protect your spine and improve your flexibility. Getting down to the correct level improves things instantly, and makes your task much easier to perform. It's a similar story when lifting objects off a high shelf: if you strain to reach up to grasp something that's too high for you, you'll become unbalanced and create tension in the muscles. It's far better to use a sturdy set of steps at home, or ask someone for assistance if you're in a shop or at the supermarket.

To take laundry in and out of a washing machine

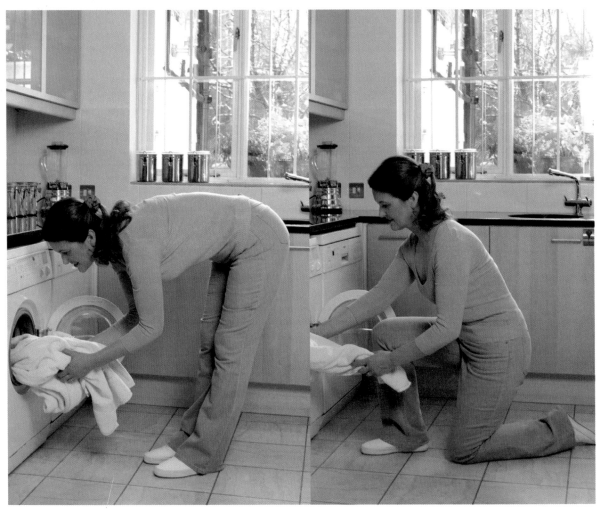

If you stand in front of the washing machine and lock your knees, you'll strain the muscles in your neck and spine. You may also find it hard to clearly see all the laundry in the drum of the machine.

Bend your knees so that you are down at the level of the washing machine. You can go down on one knee, if it helps. When you stand up, use your legs to push yourself up again. Keep your spine straight – don't let it curve forward.

To lift and carry goods from shelves

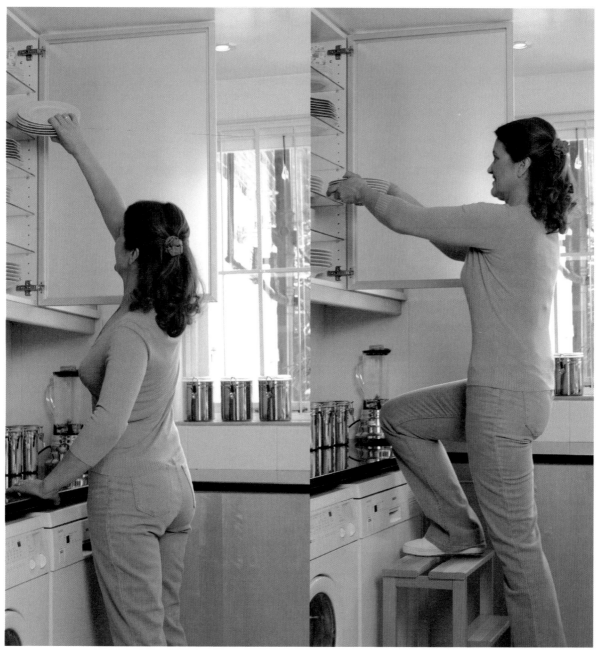

Avoid the temptation to reach up to a high shelf for something and, in the process, strain your muscles.

Position a set of steps, or a stool with fold-out steps, against the kitchen units and directly below the shelf. Step up until you are at eye level with the shelf. Ensure that your feet are flat and firmly positioned on the step. Bend your elbows a little, keep your shoulder blades down, and lean forward slightly to grasp the objects. Then step carefully back down.

Car journeys

Getting into the car

If you have problems with your joints, getting into and out of cars can be tricky. However, the method described here is not just for the stiff and elderly; girls wearing mini skirts would be well advised to use it as well.

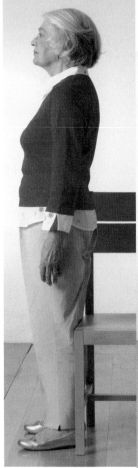

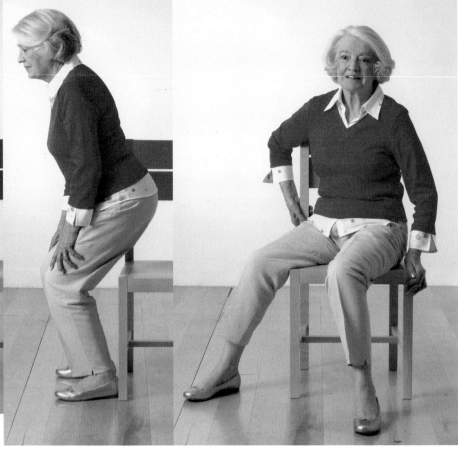

1 Stand with your back to the side of the car seat.

2 Engage your stomach muscles and lean forward from the waist. Put your hands on your thighs and lower your bottom toward the seat.

3 Sit down on the car seat, placing your right hand on the back of the seat, and your left hand on the front of the seat.

Lean back toward the far-side seat and swing your legs round into the car, using your stomach muscles and your hands to help you. Sit up straight, with your hands on the steering wheel if you are in the driver's seat.

After hip surgery, physios often recommend that you place a plastic bag on the car seat to make it easier to swivel round. Anyone who has trouble getting into or out of a car might find this tip helpful.

THE PILATES LIFESTYLE

Getting out of the car

To get out, simply reverse the procedure for getting in.

1. Swivel round and swing your legs out of the car door, while leaning back toward the seat beside you.

2. Once your feet are on the ground, bend forward from the waist, keeping your back straight, then use your muscles to pitch your weight upright.

While driving

If you are the driver, adjust your seat carefully so that you can hold the steering wheel with your upper arms by your sides and your elbows bent at right angles. Your hips and knees should also be at right angles, with the pedals within easy reach. Make sure that you can see into the rear-view mirror without stretching, leaning, or turning your head.

Automatic cars are not so good for you because the left foot sits idle while the right foot does all the work, so you will have a tendency to lean into your left hip. You shouldn't have a problem using a gear lever if your seat is in the correct position.

While you are driving, use your stomach muscles to keep your back straight instead of letting it slump into an S shape. Keep your shoulders relaxed; it's easy for them to tighten up, especially if traffic is stressful and you're late for an appointment.

Whenever you stop at traffic lights, use the rest period to exercise and ease out any tension. Put on the handbrake and rest your right leg. Shrug your shoulders to your ears and let them drop down. Think of sliding your shoulder blades down your back. Turn your head slowly to the left and then the right. Pull your stomach toward the back of the seat. Squeeze your glutes and, finally, point and flex each foot.

CAUTION: If you are prone to lower back pain, buy a specially designed lumbar cushion or back rest to support your back when you're driving.

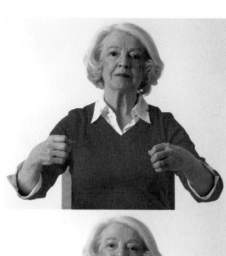
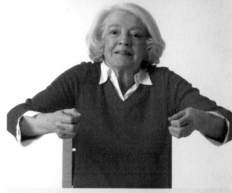
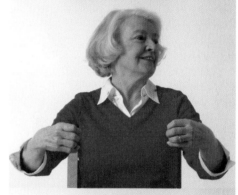
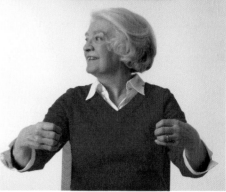

WESTCHESTER PUBLIC LIBRARY CHESTERTON, IN

Doing housework

Housework isn't designed to be done by people with bad backs, hips, knees, or elbows. There are too many tasks that encourage awkward twisting, bending, stretching at an angle or lifting heavy weights. It can be easy for even the most able-bodied of people to injure themselves. Once you have been practising Pilates for a few weeks and have strengthened your core muscles (stomach, glutes, thighs), it will be easier for you to keep your centre of balance in the right place while you are cleaning. Done correctly, household chores can provide a mini-workout that's good for you. Here are the right – and wrong – ways to do three common tasks.

Ironing

DON'T hunch your shoulders and upper back over a board that is too low for you. As well as straining your back, this action will force you to lean into your arms and hands, making it more difficult to move the iron across the fabric. Don't try to finish a large load of ironing in one go; take a break, move around, and stretch before continuing the task.

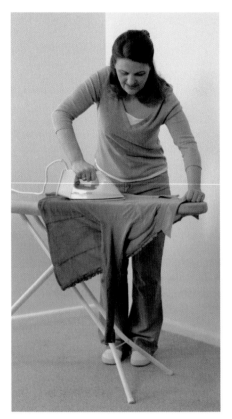

Washing dishes

DON'T curve your upper back forwards over the sink as you scrub the pots, or twist sideways to balance them in the draining rack. If you use a dishwasher, take care not to bend and twist when loading and unloading.

DO stand straight, with your stomach muscles and glutes lightly engaged. Step forward with one leg and bend the knee slightly, then lean over from the waist to reach down into the sink. Straighten up before you turn to place items in the rack to dry.

DO adjust the ironing board to the right height so that you can work with your back straight. If you are right-handed, turn your left foot out slightly to help you balance as you push the iron. If you are left-handed, turn your right foot out. Or, if you prefer, you can iron sitting down with the board adjusted to a height that allows you to work easily with your upper arms by your sides and your elbows bent at right angles.

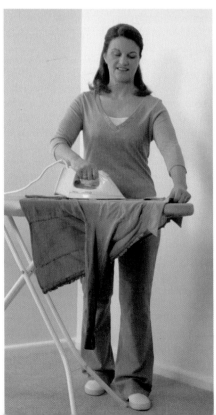

Vacuuming

DON'T bend over with straight legs, or lean right over to try to push the vacuum cleaner under a chair or into a hard-to-reach area. Cylinder vacuum cleaners can be harder to manipulate than upright ones, as there's a tendency for people to bend over to operate them.

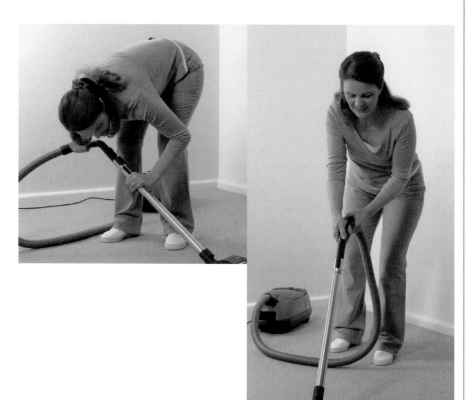

DO stand with one foot in front of the other and the knee slightly bent to take your weight as you push forward. Hold your stomach muscles in. Breathe out as you use your body weight (not just your arms) to push the cleaner away from you. Breathe in as you pull the vacuum cleaner back. If you need to vacuum under a piece of furniture, get down on one knee to reach, rather than bending over.

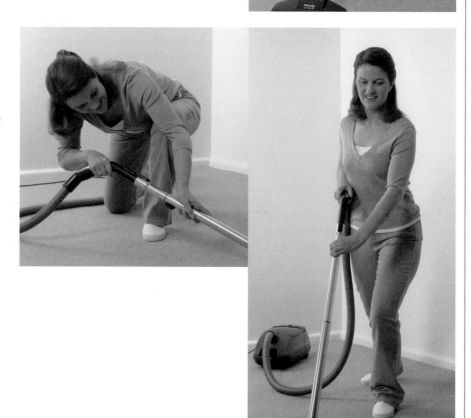

43

Aerobic exercise

The differences between aerobic and anaerobic exercise are bio-chemical. Without getting too technical, aerobic exercise allows the muscles to work at a steady pace by pushing your heart and breathing rate up to supply plenty of oxygen-rich blood to the muscles. Anaerobic exercise works individual muscles more intensively without increasing the heart rate, so it can't be sustained for a long period. Both forms of exercise are essential for good health and fitness levels because aerobic exercise gives your heart and lungs a workout and burns off calories, while anaerobic exercise tones, strengthens, and lengthens muscles.

Pilates is anaerobic, so you should supplement the workouts with your choice of aerobic exercise, perhaps alternating them on different days. Choose whatever you enjoy, so long as it doesn't aggravate existing joint or health conditions. You can use what you learn in Pilates to exercise safely and without risk of injury. Here's some specific advice on aerobic exercise.

Cycling

Choose a bicycle that has the seat, handlebars, and pedals at the correct distance from each other so that you are not hunched over, or straining your legs to fully extend the pedals. When stationary, both feet should just touch the ground. If you do a lot of cycling, the calves and the "quad" muscles at the fronts of your thighs can become over-strong. You should compensate by doing lots of hamstring exercises, and calf and quad stretches in your Pilates workouts.

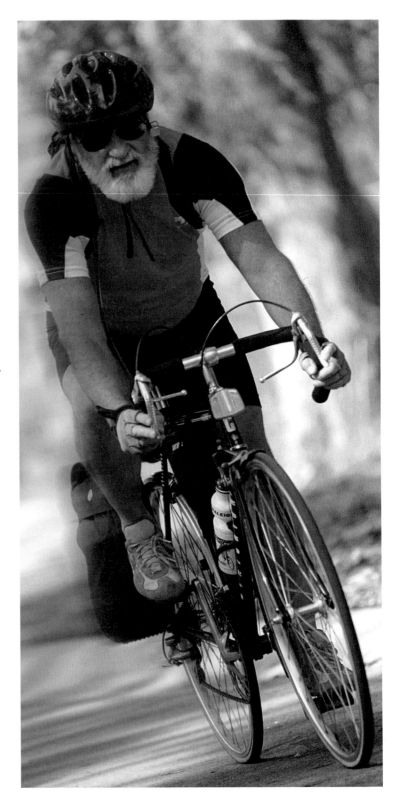

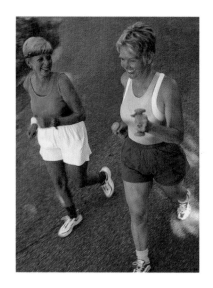

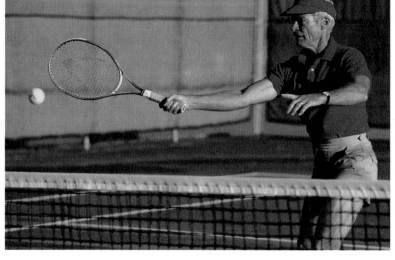

Brisk walking

Wear comfortable, supportive, low-heeled shoes that will allow the feet to bend fully. If the soles are too thick or inflexible, you will strain your lower leg muscles. Walk from the heel through to the toes, keeping your back straight, your shoulders relaxed, and your stomach muscles and glutes lightly engaged.

Running

This sport is not suitable for anyone with knee, hip, or neck problems. If you like running, make sure that you buy properly sprung shoes that absorb most of the shock of your feet hitting the ground, instead of transmitting it up through your bones.

Racquet sports and golf

These sports all use one side of the body more than the other, so it's important to counteract the imbalance in the rest of your exercise regime by doing more repetitions of the appropriate exercises on the less-used side. If you are feeling particularly one-sided after playing, ask someone to check whether you are holding one shoulder higher, or if your back is curving. If this is the case, it may be a good idea to go to a physio for an MOT from time to time.

Aerobic classes (and videos)

Be aware that aerobic sessions tend to concentrate on large muscle groups. You may need to compensate for this by working the opposite groups of muscles in Pilates. Aerobics instructors may show you ways of doing exercises that Pilates instructors would consider unsafe, but you can protect yourself by remembering to engage your abdominals and glutes to protect your spine, and by keeping your back straight as you work out.

Swimming

This is a wonderful exercise that is generally safe even if you have joint problems – so long as you keep your spine straight. If you arch your upper back to keep your head out of the water, this will strain your lower back before long. If you are not confident about your swimming technique, most pools offer refresher tuition to correct your strokes. Avoid any strokes that are uncomfortable, for example, breaststroke is not advisable if you have a lower back or neck problem.

Healthy eating

Although there a few good books on nutrition, bookshops are often overflowing with the latest fad diets. The basic rules about eating healthily are simple to take on board.

- Eat at least five portions of fruit and vegetables a day. A single portion is the equivalent of one medium apple, a palmful of broccoli, or a bowl of salad.

- Eat fruit and vegetables of lots of different colours: red peppers, yellow corn, orange carrots, dark green kale, and so on. That way you'll get a wider range of vitamins and minerals than if you stick to bananas and garden peas day in, day out.

- Eat plenty of fibre. Choose wholemeal bread, wholegrain cereals, oats, beans, and lentils and other pulses, which all help to keep the digestive system functioning more smoothly.

- Eat food that's as fresh as possible and don't overcook it. Think of steaming and grilling rather than boiling and deep-frying.

- Cut back on empty calories – those snacks that look momentarily tempting but contain no nutritional value whatsoever.

- And avoid any diet plans that cut out a whole food group, such as very-low-carb or very-low-fat diets. We need nutrients from every food group to keep us healthy.

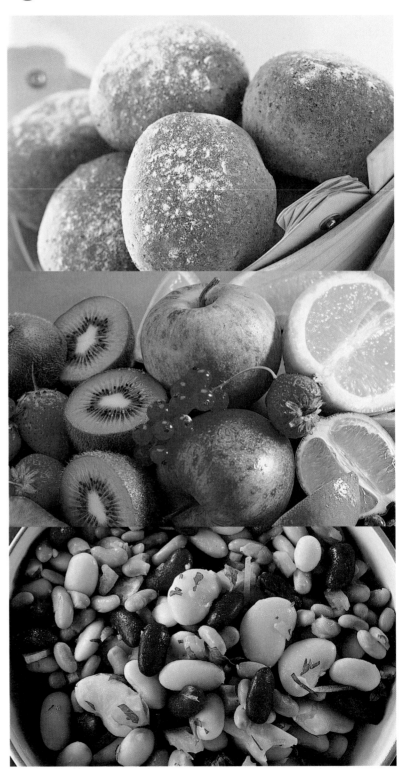

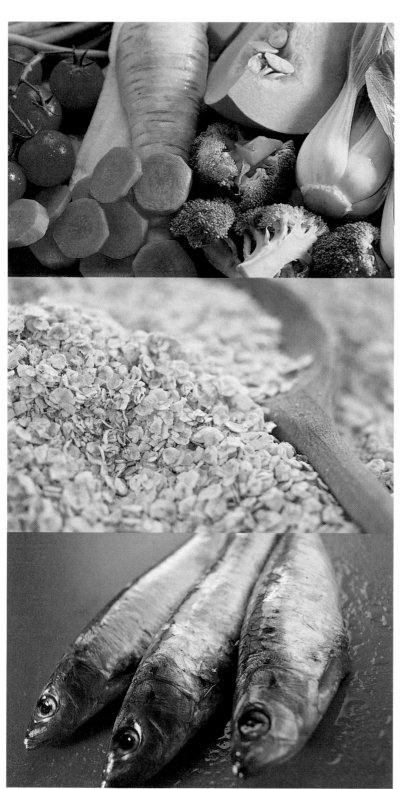

Supplements

As well as eating good-quality food, I often recommend a few supplements to those who are over 50.

- Glucosamine sulphate is remarkably effective in helping to repair stiff, painful, and damaged joints, so you should definitely give it a try if you have arthritis, back pain, or you sustain any joint injuries.

- A vitamin D supplement with calcium can help people with osteoporosis (or its precursor, osteopenia), and can reduce the risk of bones fracturing.

- A daily multivitamin and mineral supplement can be beneficial, but make sure you don't exceed the recommended daily amount (RDA) of any individual nutrient. You'll find these recommendations listed on the packaging of most supplements, as well as on food packaging.

- Omega-3 fish oils can ease joint inflammation, and reduce the furring up of the arteries, therefore helping to prevent heart disease. Some experts think that they reduce the risk of certain cancers as well.

CAUTION: Consult your doctor before using supplements if you are already taking medication, or if you suspect you have a deficiency.

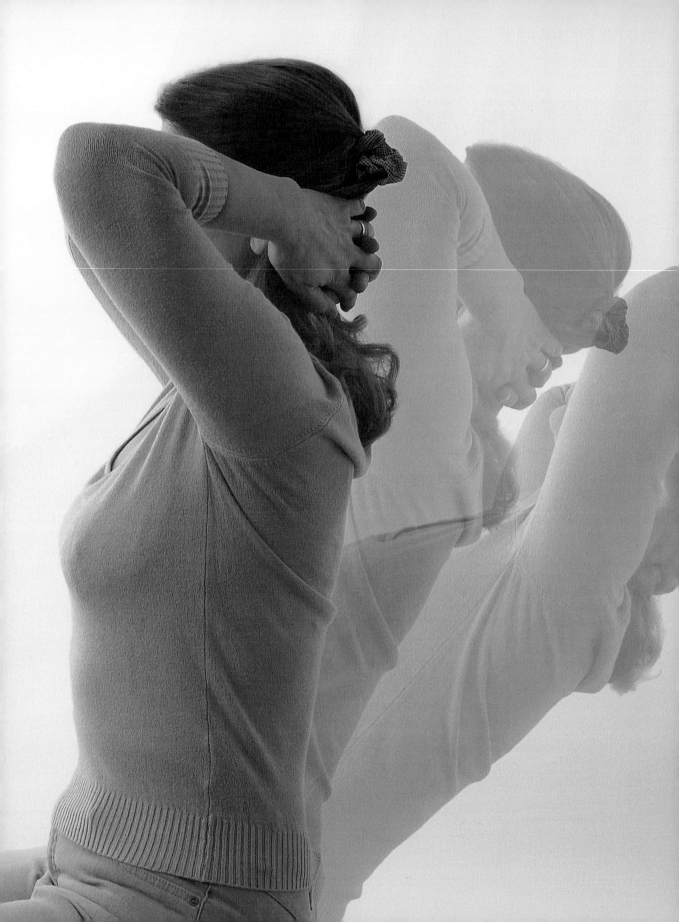

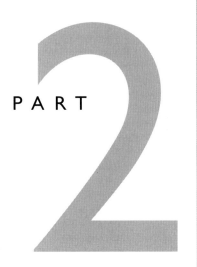

PART

2

A top-to-toe workout

In this chapter, you will find a basic Pilates work-out that uses all the main muscle groups. It will take about an hour to do the whole routine, but if you can't spare so much time you can be selective. Make a note of any exercises that you skip and try to include them during your next session in order to keep a balance in the strength of different muscles.

Wear loose, comfortable clothing without any tight belts or fastenings, and socks or bare feet rather than shoes. You will need some cushions or pillows and an upright chair without any arms. Make sure that the room is warm enough and that you can work without interruptions.

Go slowly at the beginning, concentrating on the sensations and trying to form memories of which muscles you use and what each move feels like. If this is your first-ever Pilates session and you manage to complete all the exercises, I guarantee that you will feel better afterwards!

Static abs – semi-supine

You first tried Static abs while lying on your side (see pp.22–23). To begin the Top-to-toe work-out, try doing Static abs lying on your back, which is an important starting point for many Pilates exercises. It can be harder to isolate the abdominal muscles in this position, but once you know how to control them you should find this an effective exercise.

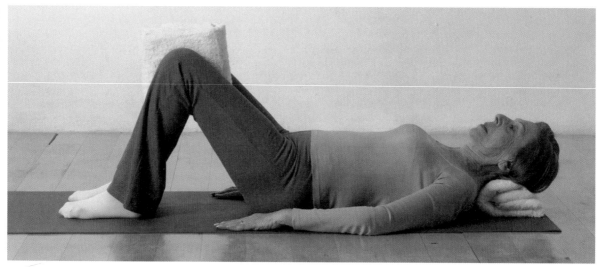

1 Lie on your back with your knees bent and feet hip-width apart (this is known as the "semi-supine" position). Place a folded towel between your knees and another under your head so that your neck and spine are straight. Relax your arms and shoulders. Breathe in.

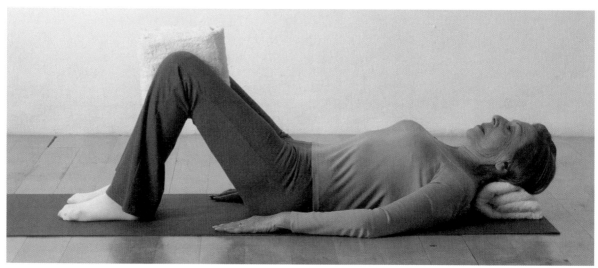

2 As you breathe out, pull your abdomen down toward the floor. Make sure that your shoulders are still relaxed.

Release, and repeat 10 times.

Pelvic tilts

This exercise is a more advanced version of the Bridge (see p.25).

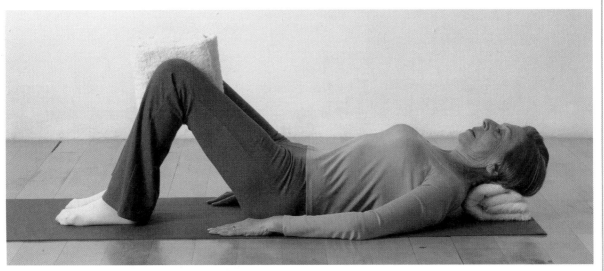

Lie on your back with your knees bent and feet hip-width apart. Place a folded towel between your knees and another towel under your head. Relax your upper body and then breathe in.

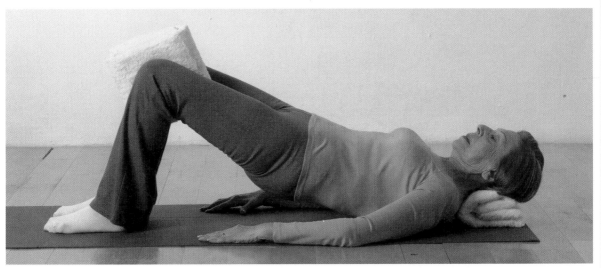

2 As you breathe out, pull your abdomen back toward the floor and lift your pelvic floor muscles. (These are a "hammock" of muscles running from the pubic bone at the front to the anus at the back. If you have trouble locating yours, read the advice on page 94.) As you lift your pelvic floor, tilt your pelvis as if you are trying to curl your tailbone round between your legs toward the front. Don't feel as though you have to go too far. Make sure you aren't squeezing your thighs together or creating tension in your upper body. The abdominal and pelvic floor muscles should be doing all the work. Breathe in.

Breathe out as you slowly roll your pelvis back down to the ground again. Repeat 10 times.

CAUTION: If you have lordosis – a pronounced arch in your lower back – try doing this exercise with your lower legs resting on a low chair. If you have kyphosis – a forward curve in the upper back – support your head and shoulders with cushions so that they feel comfortable and are not forced down into the floor as you exercise.

51

Leg slides

There are two ways of doing this exercise: with, or without, a stool. Use the version with a stool (see opposite) if you are prone to lower back pain. Those who don't have back problems might like to try both versions because they work slightly different areas of abdominal muscle.

I Lie on your back with your knees bent and feet hip-width apart. Place your hands on your lower stomach, just above your hip bones. Breathe in.

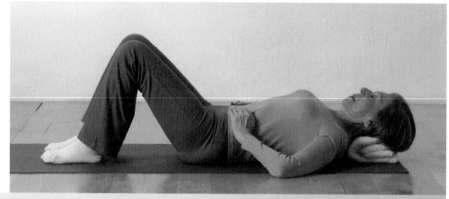

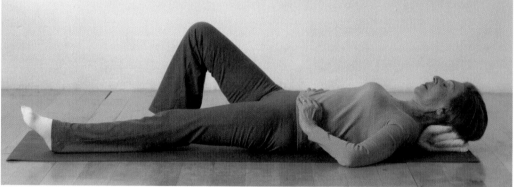

2 As you breathe out, pull your abdominals back to the floor, squeeze your left buttock, and slide your left heel away from you, but without letting your pelvis move. Concentrate on keeping the pelvis in exactly the same position; only slide your leg as far as it can go without tilting the pelvis. Your abdominal muscles should be controlling the movement; if you feel strain in the right leg, try the version with the stool. Don't force your leg straight – just go as far as feels comfortable. Breathe in.

Breathe out and return the left leg to the starting position. Repeat 10 times with each leg.

Variation

As you slide your leg, raise the opposite arm up over your head and behind you until your arm is by your ear and your palm faces the ceiling. As you slide your leg back, rest your arm by your side. Repeat with the other leg and arm.

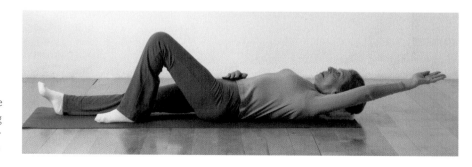

Leg slides with stool

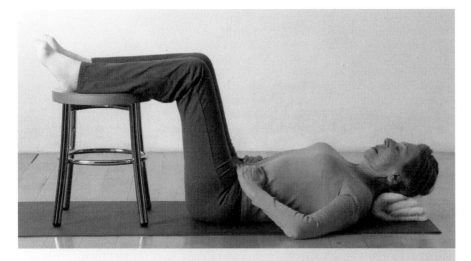

1 Position a low stool in front of you and lie on your back. The stool should of a height that when you rest your lower legs on it, your hips and knees are at right angles. Support your neck with a folded towel, place your hands on your lower stomach just above the hip bones, and relax your shoulders into the floor. Breathe in.

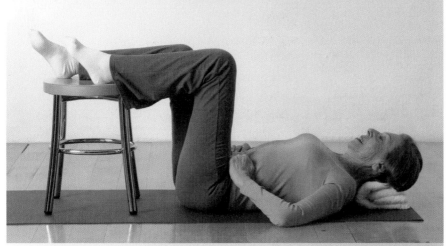

2 As you breathe out, engage your stomach muscles and slide your left heel toward you. Don't let your back arch. Keep the pelvis still and breathe in.

Breathe out and slide your left heel back to the starting position.

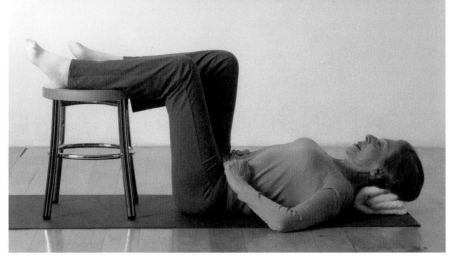

3 Breathe out, engage your abdominals, and slide your right heel toward you.

Repeat the movement 10 times with each leg.

53

Adductor squeeze

In this exercise, you are going to learn to isolate the inner thigh muscles. You may feel your glutes engaging as well, but keep your concentration focused on the inner thighs and learn how to make these muscles work.

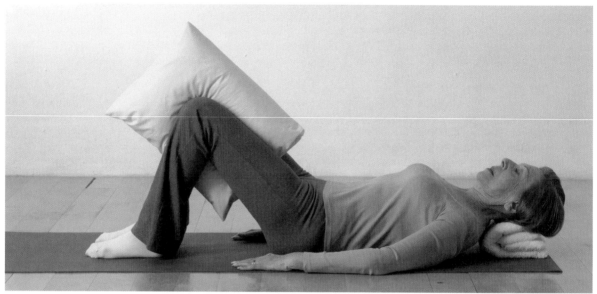

1 Lie on your back with your knees bent and feet hip-width apart. Place a pillow between your knees and a folded towel under your head to support your neck. Relax your upper body into the floor. Breathe in.

2 As you breathe out, engage your abdominals and then pull your inner thighs together so that you gently squeeze the pillow. Don't grip too hard.

Hold for four seconds, then release. Repeat 10 times.

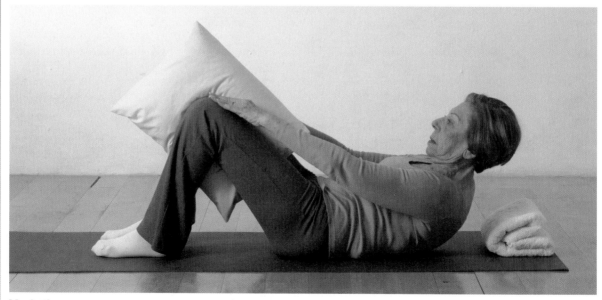

Variation
As you pull your inner thighs together and gently squeeze the pillow, slide your hands up to your knees, draw your abs in, lift your chin up, and look straight ahead. Hold for four seconds, then release slowly.

Upper body release

This is a good exercise for loosening up tight shoulder blades. If you're in the office and there's room to lie down, you could try this exercise in the middle of a working day.

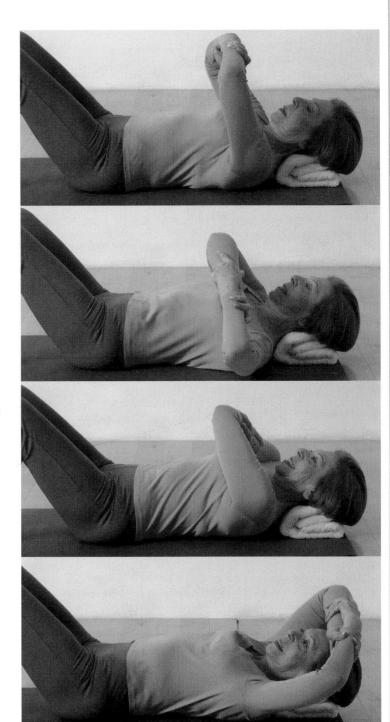

1 Lie on your back with your knees bent, feet hip-width apart, and a folded towel supporting your head. Relax your shoulders, then clasp your forearms in front of your breastbone. If this feels too tight, you could try placing one hand on top of the other, or touching your fingertips together or holding an object such as a tape or CD. Breathe in.

2 As you breathe out, engage your abdominals and circle your arms round to the left. You'll feel your shoulder blades moving underneath you and the muscles between them will release. If they are particularly tight, you might hear a bit of gravelly crunching as they loosen.

3 Continue to circle your arms up toward the top of your head, keeping your forearms in a straight line. Breathe in.

4 Breathe out and circle your arms round to the right.

Breathe in to return to the centre. Repeat 10 times on each side.

Variation
Allow your arms to stretch even further as you circle them so that your elbows touch the floor briefly.

Side-lying static abs

Although you have tried this exercise already (see pp.22–23), it needs to be repeated in this Top-to-toe workout because it uses a different part of the abdominal muscles than the semi-supine Static abs (see p.50). It also prepares you for the outer thigh exercise that follows.

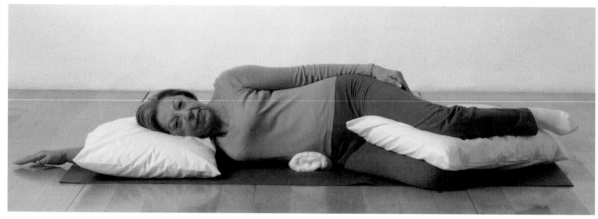

Lie on your right side and extend your right arm. Curl your knees up. Place a pillow between your thighs and another under your head. Place a folded towel under your waist to support the spine. Rest your hand on your hip. Breathe in and let your stomach hang down toward the floor.

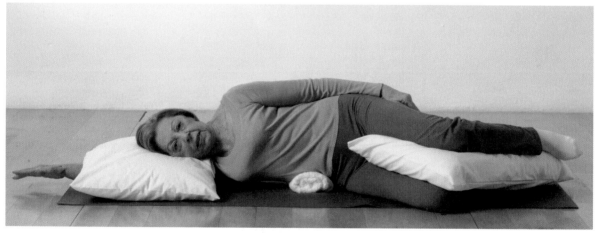

2 Breathe out and pull your stomach up first, and then backward.

Repeat 10 times on each side.

Outer thigh lifts

Once you get into position for this exercise, take a minute to check your alignment because the movements won't be as effective if you are even just one centimetre out. If necessary, find a piece of furniture or a wall to lie against to ensure that your back is straight.

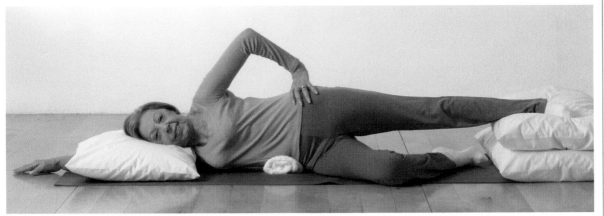

1 Lie on your right side with your right arm extended and a pillow under your head. Bend your right leg to try to create right angles at the hip and the knee. Place a couple of pillows underneath your left foot, and a folded towel under your waist so that your spine doesn't sink down to the floor. Rest the fingers of your left hand on your left hip.

Before you proceed to step 2, run through this checklist:
- Are your hip bones directly in line with each other?
- Are your shoulder joints directly in line with each other?
- Is your spine in a straight line, and not dipping at the waist or in the neck?

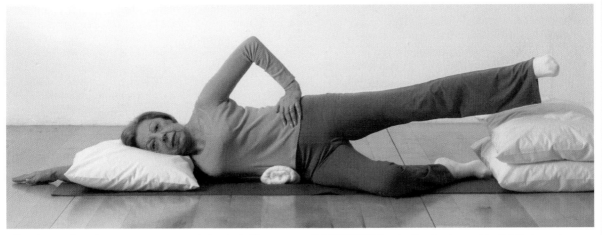

2 As you breathe out, engage your abdominals. Flex your left foot, stretch down through the heel, and lift the left leg without moving your hips. Don't try to lift too far; the benefit is in the first few centimetres.

CAUTION: Look after the lower hip: if it feels uncomfortable, adjust your angle or place a cushion under it, or both. Avoid this exercise after a hip replacement operation until you are free of pain.

Return to the start position. Repeat five times on each side.

Lying glute squeezes

It's harder to contract the glute muscles when you're lying down than when you're standing up. If you can't manage this exercise at first, keep

practising standing glute squeezes (see p.24) and try these lying glute squeezes again in a week.

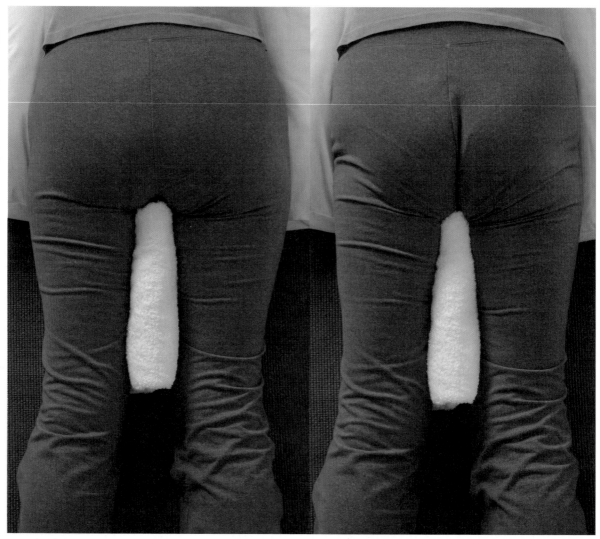

I Lie face down on the floor with a folded towel between your thighs. Place a pillow under your abdomen and rest your forehead and your hands on another folded towel. If this feels uncomfortable in your upper back, try slipping a small cushion under each shoulder. When you're ready, breathe in.

2 As you breathe out, squeeze your buttocks towards each other. You should feel the stomach muscles engage and your lower back gently lengthen. Don't let your legs turn inward.

Hold the squeeze for four seconds. Repeat 10 times.

Hamstring curls

It's very important that you raise your leg in a straight line for this exercise. Ask someone to watch you doing it and correct you if necessary.

Or imagine a line that runs directly between your heel and your fingertips on each side, and don't waver from it.

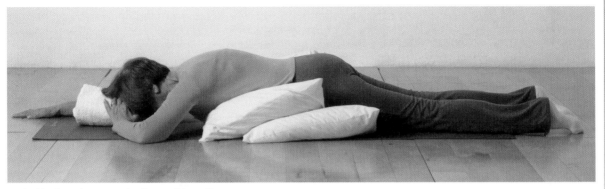

1 Lie face down on the floor with a pillow or two under your abdomen. Rest your forehead and left hand on a folded towel. Extend your right hand out along the floor by your head. Stretch into each leg a little to make sure that they are straight and parallel. Breathe in.

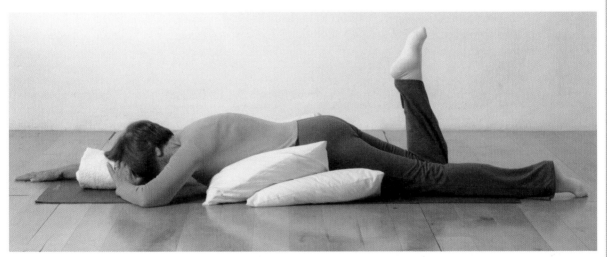

2 As you breathe out, very slowly bend your right leg until your knee is at a right angle. Imagine your right heel runs in a straight line towards your right fingers. Don't jerk, and keep your foot soft. You should be able to feel the muscles in the back of your thigh working.

Breathe in to lower your right leg to the ground. Repeat 10 times with each leg.

CAUTION: If you find that your leg jerks or shakes while doing this exercise, try making the movement smaller. One way to do this is to place a cushion under your feet and lift from a raised position. Those with knee problems might find it helps if you place a folded towel under each thigh so that your knees aren't pushed into the floor. If you experience any discomfort, just stop.

The Arrow

This exercise gives a great stretch to the upper back as you slide your shoulder blades down and lengthen your neck away from your body.

CAUTION: You may find this exercise uncomfortable if you suffer from back or neck pain, or kyphosis. Don't worry about it – do the sitting lats exercise on page 63 for now, and try this exercise again in a few weeks.

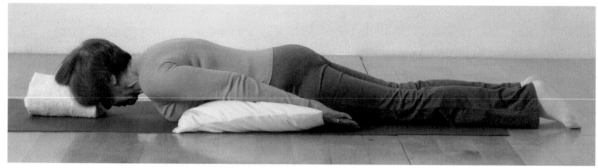

I Lie on your front with your abdomen supported by a pillow and your forehead resting on a folded towel. Place a cushion under each shoulder if you find it helps you to relax your upper back. Rest your arms by your sides. Your legs should be hip-width apart and the heels turned slightly inward. Breathe in.

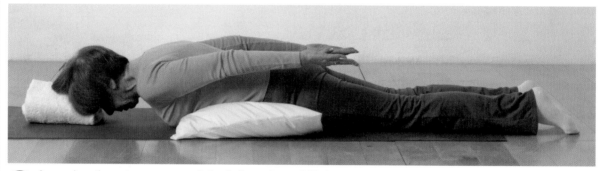

2 As you breathe out, engage your abdominal muscles and lift the palms of your hands upward, to about the level of your bottom. Keep resting your head on the towel. Feel the stretch.

Breathe in to return to the starting position. Repeat 10 times.

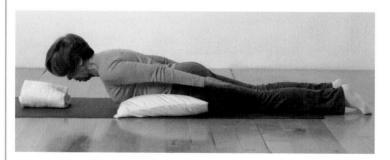

Variation
As you lift the palms of your hands upward, try sliding your shoulder blades down your back and lifting your head and breastbone, stretching them forward. Keep your upper spine in a straight line and don't bend your head back.

Back stretch

Always do this back stretch after the Arrow. It's a good way to finish off any exercises that involve lying on the floor before moving on to the next part of your routine.

CAUTION: Be careful not to strain your knees as you sit back onto your heels.

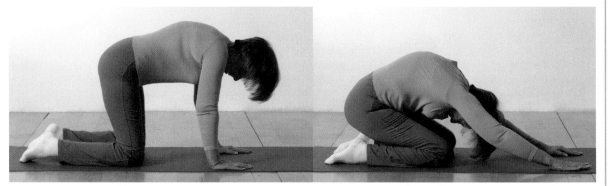

1 From lying on your stomach, place your hands just in front of your shoulders and push up so that you are kneeling on all fours. Drop your head down to relax your neck. Breathe in.

2 As you breathe out, engage your abdominals and slide your hands forward as far as you can while lowering your bottom back to your heels.

Hold for 10 seconds.

Sitting glute stretch

You have used your buttocks and hips for several exercises so far in this Top-to-toe workout, so take the time now to sit on a chair and stretch your glute muscles properly.

1 Sit upright on a chair. Lift your left leg and cross it over your right leg so that your left ankle rests on your right knee. Keep your left knee open and your left hand resting on your knee. Breathe in. As you exhale, lean forward. Keep your back as straight as possible. Let your hand push your left knee gently down.

Hold for four seconds. Then repeat with the other leg.

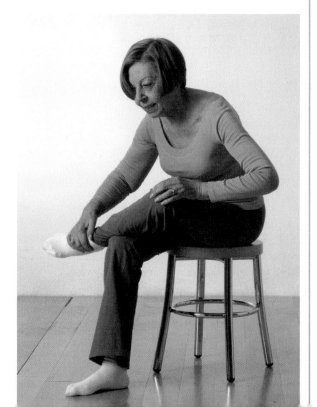

Shoulder shrugs

Try to practise shoulder shrugs as often as you remember to do them. Although it's a simple exercise, it's effective at releasing the tension that builds up in the neck and upper back.

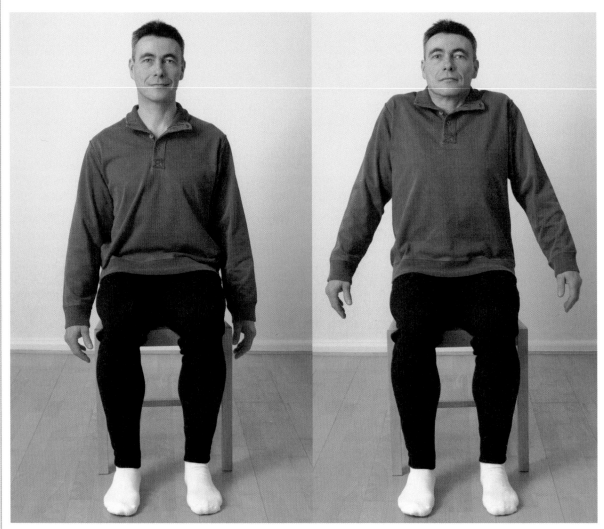

1 Sit upright on a chair with your back well supported. Relax your shoulders down and let your arms and hands hang loosely at your sides.

2 Shrug your shoulders right up toward your ears. Let your arms remain dangling. Then relax your shoulders back down again.

Repeat five times.

Sitting lats

The muscles you used to slide your shoulder blades down your back in the Arrow (see p.60) are the latissimus dorsi muscles (we'll call them lats, for short). They should control most arm movements, but when these muscles are weak people tend to use their shoulder muscles instead. By strengthening the lats you can release any upper back tension and loosen bunched-up muscles in the shoulders.

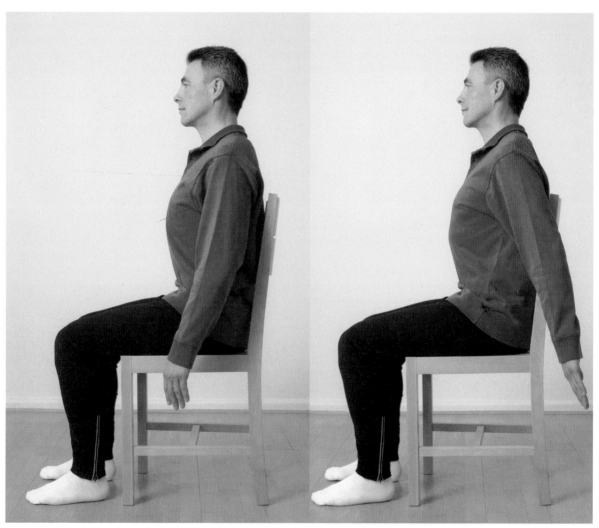

1 Sit on a stool or chair without arms. Your hips and knees should be at right angles when your feet are flat on the floor. Let your arms and hands hang loosely by your sides.

2 Face your palms backward and very slightly outward. As you breathe out, engage your abdominals and push your left palm back. You shouldn't feel any tension in your shoulders; the lats will be doing the work, and you should be able to feel them just beneath the shoulder blades.

Breathe in and return your left arm to your side. Repeat five times with each arm, then repeat the exercise five times with both arms together.

Working the upper torso

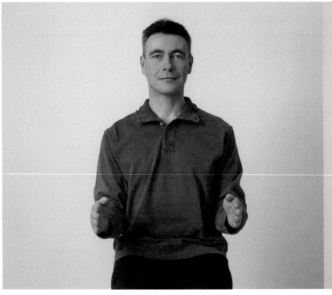

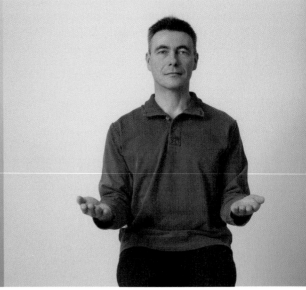

1 Sit on a chair or stool with your elbows bent at right angles, your upper arms by your sides, your lower arms out in front of you, and with your palms facing inward. Check that your shoulders are relaxed. Breathe in.

3 Move your lower arms back until they are in front of you. Turn your palms upward, still keeping your elbows by your sides.

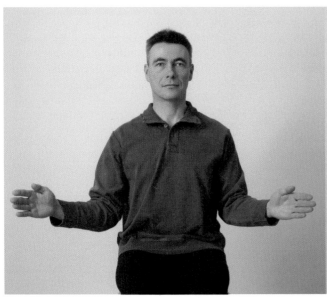

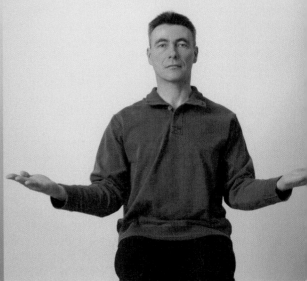

2 As you breathe out, engage your abdominals, and open your lower arms out to the sides. You will feel your chest opening out.

4 As you breathe out, open your arms out to the side.

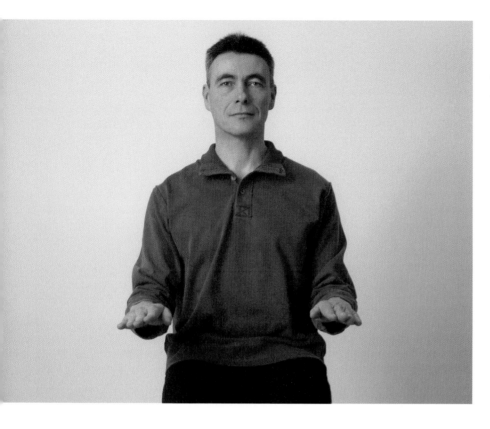

5 Move your lower arms back until they are in front of you. Turn your palms over so that they face downward.

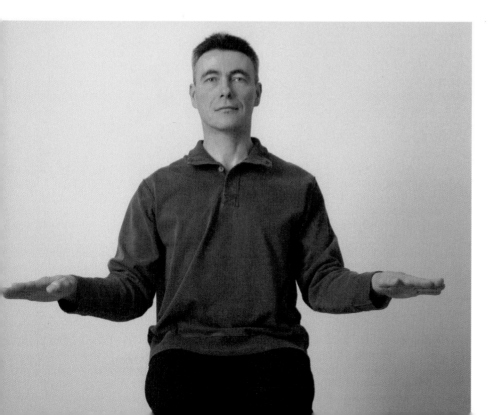

6 As you breathe out, open your arms out to the sides, feeling the shoulder blades gently pull together.

Repeat the whole sequence slowly 10 times.

TOP-TO-TOE WORKOUT

65

Cossack Arms

You tried a version of this exercise on page 33. It's useful for keeping rotational flexibility in the spine, but it can be difficult at first to stop yourself from using the neck and shoulder muscles in the movement. Concentrate on using the lats and keeping your neck and shoulders loose.

1 Sit upright on a chair or stool and touch your fingertips together in front of your breastbone. Breathe in. Breathe out, engage your abdominals, slide your shoulder blades down. Turn your upper body to the right, keeping your spine straight. Your arms should slide round softly and easily.

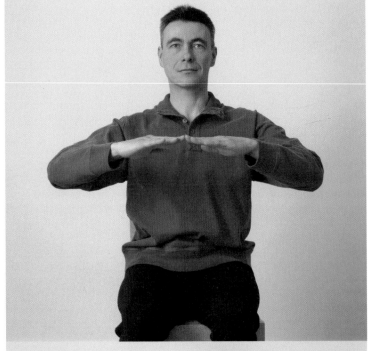

2 When you have turned as far as you can go, pause. As you breathe out turn a little further and you'll feel an extra little pull in the lats. Breathe in and return to the centre.

Repeat five times in each direction.

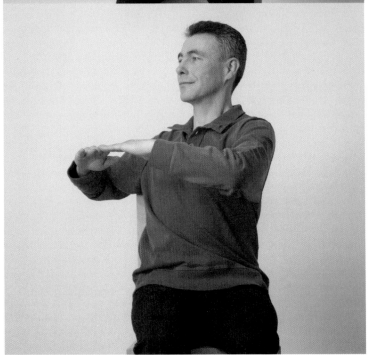

Side bends

You have tried a version of this exercise before (see p.33), but this time you'll be using a chair with a straight back and sitting side on. The chairback provides an anchor to stop you stretching too far. Use a ladderback chair or any firm, armless chair.

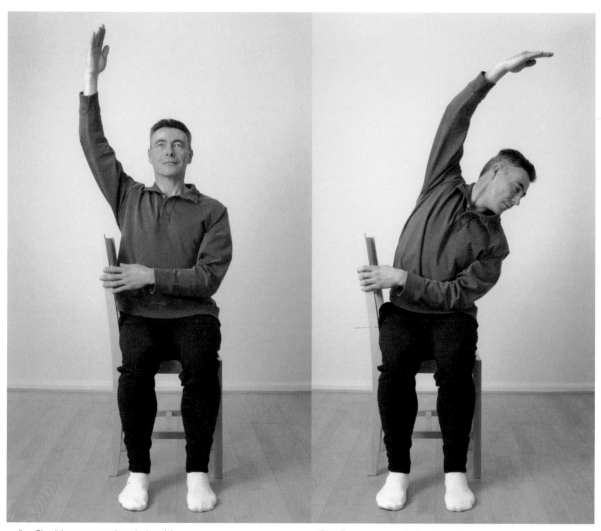

1 Sit sideways on the chair, with the back of the chair to your right side. Hold onto the back of the chair with your left hand. Your thighs should be parallel to the floor and your feet hip-width apart. Raise your right arm in a gentle curve over your head. Breathe in.

2 Engage your abdominals, turn your head to the left and bend your upper body to the left. Your right hand will limit the amount of the stretch. Breathe in to return to the centre.

Repeat five times on each side.

CAUTION: If you find it uncomfortable holding your arm up in the air, place your raised hand on the back of your head.

Inner thighs – sitting

The Adductor squeeze (see p.54) helped you to isolate the inner thigh muscles. Now try to find the same muscles in this exercise, and don't let the stronger quad muscles at the front of the thighs take over.

1 Sit on the floor with your back resting lightly against a wall or a piece of furniture. Make sure that your lower back touches the wall. Spread your legs wide.

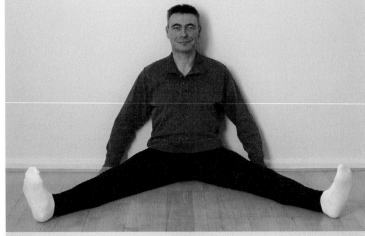

2 Bend your right leg and hold the knee with your right hand. Flex your left foot. Breathe in.

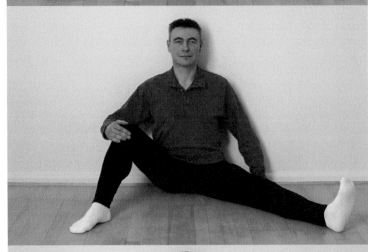

3 As you breathe out, engage your abdominals, and slide your left leg across the floor toward the bent leg. Take it past the centre line (unless you have a hip replacement, in which case you should stop at the centre line). Breathe in to return to the starting position.

Repeat five times on each leg.

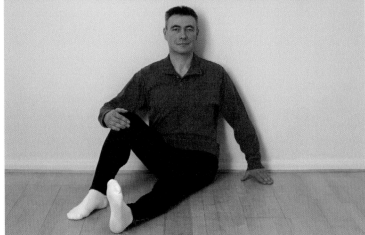

Hip roll

This exercise also uses the abdominal muscles effectively. It is a good way of releasing any lower back tension.

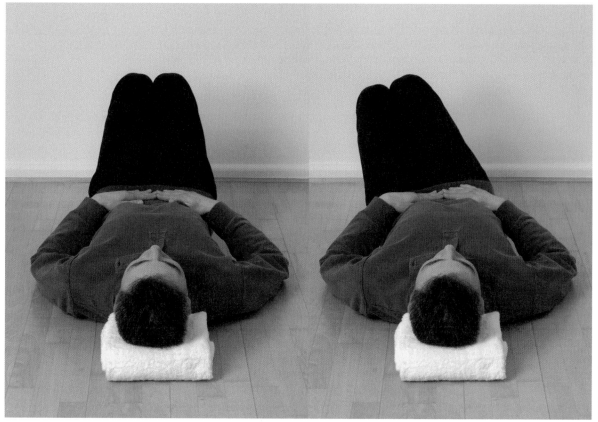

1 Lie on your back in the semi-supine position with your knees together. Place a folded towel under your head. Relax your shoulders into the floor and place your hands on your abdomen, just above your hip bones. Then breathe in.

2 As you breathe out, engage your abdominal muscles and move your knees to the left, without letting your hips move off the floor. Place your hands on the muscles just above the hips and use them to counterbalance the knee movement. It's a very small movement and should be done very slowly.

Repeat 10 times on each side.

CAUTION: If you have recently had a hip replacement, the inner thigh stretch and hip roll should be approached with caution. See page 96 for more specific advice.

Back stretch

CAUTION: If you have recently had a hip replacement, repeat the back stretch on page 61 instead of doing this stretch. See page 96 for more specific advice.

1 Lie on your back with your knees bent. Place a folded towel under your head. Relax your arms on the floor and breathe in.

2 As you breathe in, engage your abdominals and lift the right knee up towards your chest. Hold onto it with your right hand, feeling the stretch in your lower back. Your right thigh should be at right angles to the floor.

3 Keeping your right knee at your chest, raise your left knee as well and hold both knees so that they are parallel, but slightly apart. Breathe in.

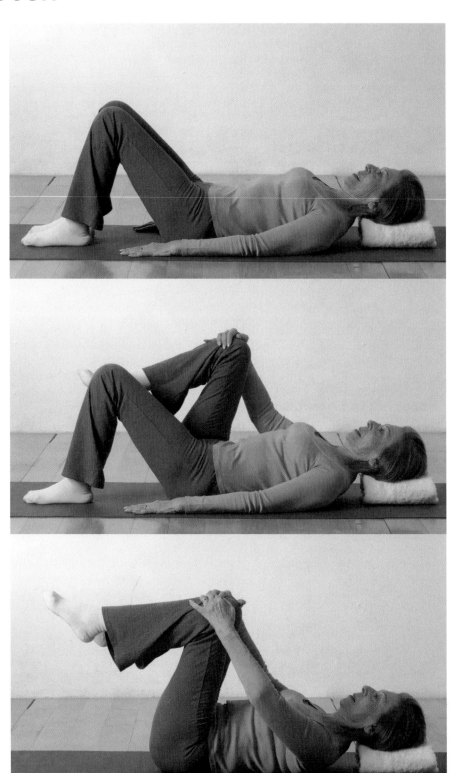

4 As you breathe out, gently pull your right knee towards your chest. Breathe in to relax, then release your right knee a little. Keep your shoulders soft.

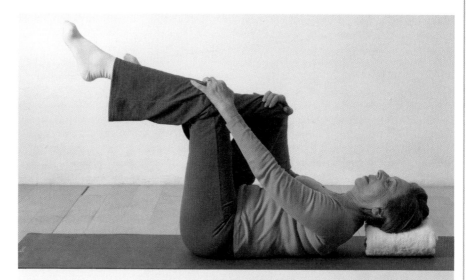

5 Breathe out, engage your abdominals, and pull the left knee toward your chest. Breathe in to relax, then release the left knee a little.

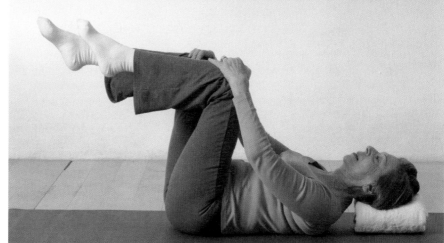

6 Breathe out and pull both knees together toward your chest (not shown). Lengthen the back of your neck. Press your knees together and imagine that you are lying on a clock face. Then slowly circle your knees four times in a clockwise direction, and four times anticlockwise. Breathe easily throughout.

Lower your right leg to the floor first, then let your left leg follow it.

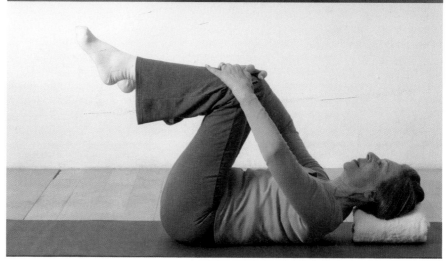

71

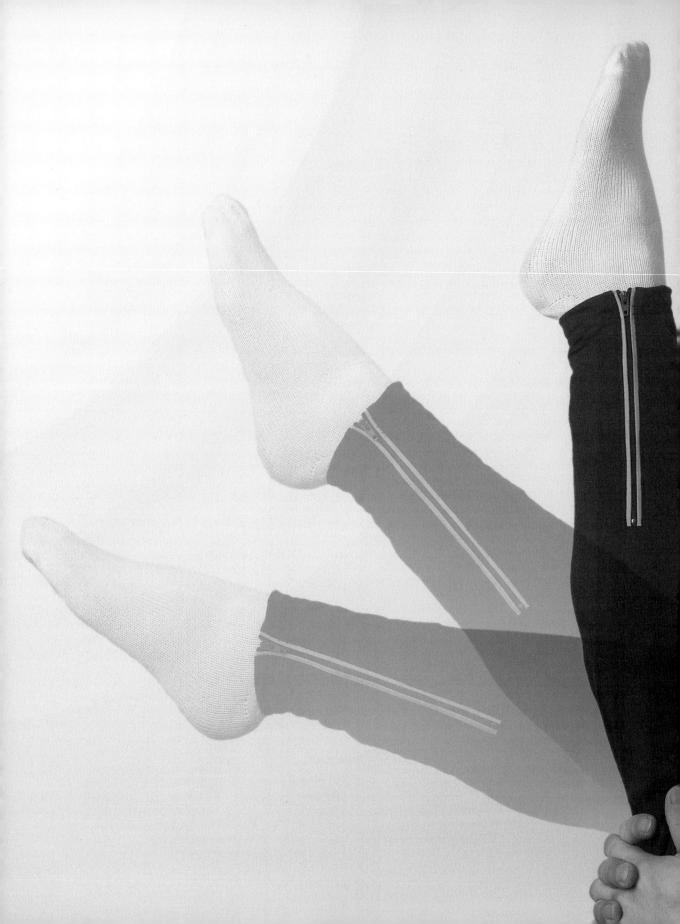

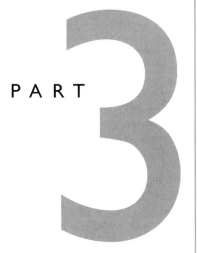

PART

3

Exercises to ease problem areas

Unlike most other exercise systems, Pilates never tries to impose a one-size-fits-all regime. We each have our own strong and weak areas, postural imbalances, and health patterns, and if we take account of them when we design an exercise programme, it can help to rectify them. You can work to make weak muscles stronger, to straighten your posture, and to improve your general balance and flexibility by selecting the appropriate exercises and doing them in the recommended way.

Read through the advice that applies to any health conditions you may suffer from, and take note of those exercises you should emphasize, and those that you should avoid. Whether you just wake up with a stiff neck some mornings or you have a serious, degenerative illness affecting your joints, you'll find some exercises in this chapter to help ease out the affected areas.

Warning

If you are being treated by a doctor or physiotherapist, I suggest that you show them this book and ask them to tick the exercises that would be safe for you to do. Avoid any that they don't recommend.

Conventional medical treatment will probably focus on the specific area that has sustained an injury; Pilates, however, can help to keep your whole body toned while you heal. For example, if a physio is treating you for a shoulder or an elbow injury, follow his or her advice about the movements that are safe for your particular condition. However, continue to work on your stomach, pelvis, and legs to ensure that your posture doesn't deteriorate while the weak area mends. If one shoulder is stiff, your knee is a bit fragile, or if you have a painful corn on one foot, your centre of gravity will try to shift sideways to protect the injured area while still keeping you balanced. The problem is that your muscles then remember this posture and stick with it long after your shoulder/knee/foot has healed.

Use the exercises in this section to help your problem areas, but combine them with any of the other exercises you can manage from the Top-to-toe workout (see pp.50–71) to keep yourself as fit and as flexible as possible. If in doubt, ask a qualified Pilates teacher to explain which are the best exercises to suit your own particular needs.

Arthritis

Arthritis is actually a blanket term for a number of disorders that cause joint pain and stiffness. The causes can either be genetic or occupational. Osteoarthritis is caused by wear and tear on the cartilage that protects joints, so the bones no longer move smoothly over each other. You can have osteoarthritis in just one or two joints, while the rest are fine. Rheumatoid arthritis is a disease causing inflammation of the lining of the joints. It can affect other body systems, such as the heart and lungs, making sufferers prone to fatigue.

Pilates can be helpful for all kinds of arthritis because by learning to maintain good posture you can prevent the body twisting to protect the site of pain. Gentle exercise that takes a joint through its range of movement will help to ease stiffness and maintain mobility. Rather than trying to do longer sessions, it can be a good idea to exercise in short, 10–15-minute sessions up to twice a day. Use Pilates moves to warm-up before you try any aerobic exercise.

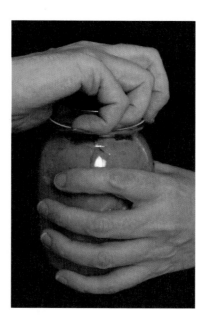

Twisting off lids

Use a grip or jar opener if you have one, otherwise hold the jar in one hand and the lid in the other. Turn your wrists in opposite directions to unscrew the lid.

CAUTION: If you have arthritis, you should avoid any strenuous movements that tire or strain the joints. Always stop if you feel any pain. When a joint is especially inflamed, the range of movement should be reduced to keep within the comfort zone. If even mild exercise is irritating the joint, rest may be needed.

Stiff hands

The joints in the hands can be particularly prone to arthritis and general stiffness. The exercises shown here help to loosen them up. Keep your hands warm at all times and try taking glucosamine sulphate supplements to see if they help. If you work on a computer keyboard, arrange your desk so that your elbows and lower arms rest on the surface of the desk. Keep your wrists as flat as possible while you type. If you have any problems with your hands or wrists, avoid exercises that require you to kneel on all fours, such as the back stretch on page 61. Alternatively, you could lean your hands onto a folded towel rather than onto the floor so that your wrists aren't bent so far back.

Releasing the wrists

Rest your forearm on the arm of a chair or the end of a table. Extend your hand over the edge. Clench your hand into a soft fist and gently move it up and down 10 times, then from side to side 10 times.

Repeat with the other hand.

CAUTION: Avoid these exercises if you have carpal tunnel syndrome or repetitive strain injury; your specialist will probably recommend that you rest your hands and wrists. However, you can still try to maintain correct posture at all times without putting any strain on the affected area.

Releasing the wrists

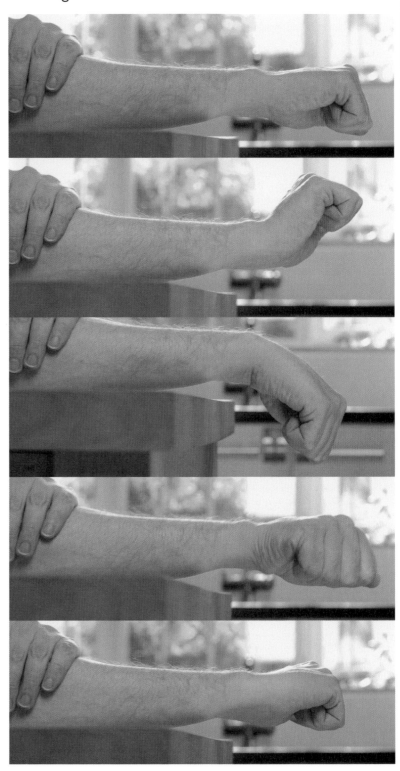

Stiff hands

Squeezing a ball

Touching your thumb

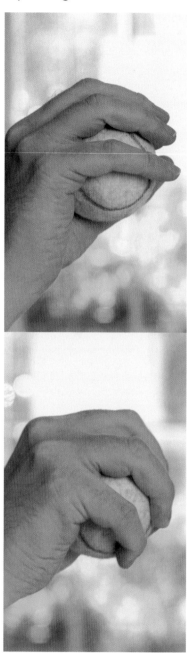

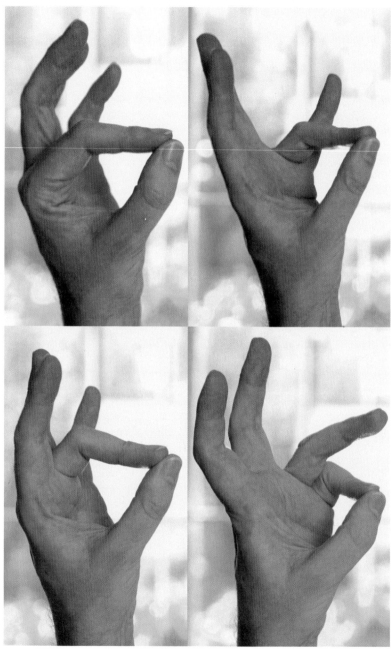

Buy a soft ball, and squeeze and release it whenever you have a spare moment. Knead some Plasticine or Play-doh if there's any lying around the house. If you don't have any of these, a normal sponge will do.

Firmly press your thumb against each of the fingers on the same hand, in turn. Repeat five times. Give it a jazz-time finish by wiggling all your fingers in the air!

Clasping your hands

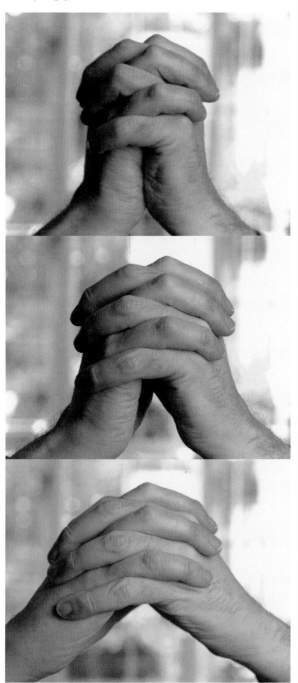

Clasp your hands together using about 50 per cent force. Try to peel them apart while resisting the movement at the same time. This is good for strengthening the muscles in the backs of the hands.

Tennis and golfer's elbow

You don't need to play tennis or golf to be afflicted with these painful conditions, caused by inflammation of the tendons that attach muscle to bone. Tennis elbow affects the muscles that straighten the fingers and wrists. It can be caused by playing tennis with a faulty grip, or any other repetitive action that tugs on the tendon attached to those muscles, such as gardening or lifting heavy objects. Golfer's elbow affects the muscles that bend the wrist and fingers. This is caused by a faulty golf grip or by gripping and twisting actions such as using a screwdriver.

The first thing to do is to stop any activity that has caused the inflammation and, when it's acute, you can apply ice packs. If it's a sports injury, get some tuition to improve your technique before you play again.

CAUTION: Avoid carrying heavy bags while you have an elbow injury, and never "lock" your elbows. If the injury has developed as a result of a particular activity, avoid it for the time being.

Frozen shoulder

Shoulder joints can become stiff and painful after an injury to the area, but sometimes they "freeze up" for no obvious reason. Frozen shoulder is the name for a condition in which the lining of the shoulder joint becomes inflamed, and there are different degrees of it. If you have a mild to moderately stiff shoulder, the exercises on these pages should help. If the pain is acute, get medical treatment. The shoulder is the most fragile joint in the human body, and the one that is hardest to fix if it gets damaged.

Arm circles

1 Stand beside a chair with your right foot in front of your left foot and your right hand holding the chair back. Bend forward from the hips, letting your left arm hang loosely down and dropping your head.

2 Circle your left arm in a clockwise direction three or four times, then reverse the movement and circle in an anticlockwise direction a few times.

Change position and repeat with the right arm.

CAUTION: Don't try to circle your arms right around the joint. Only exercise within the range of movement that feels comfortable and don't let your shoulder "click".

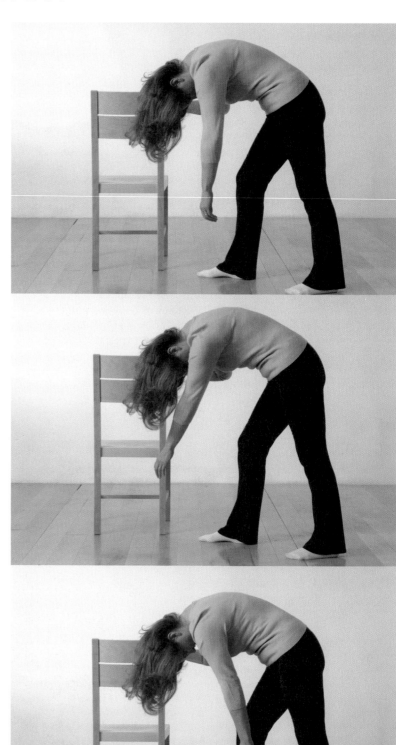

Elbow circles

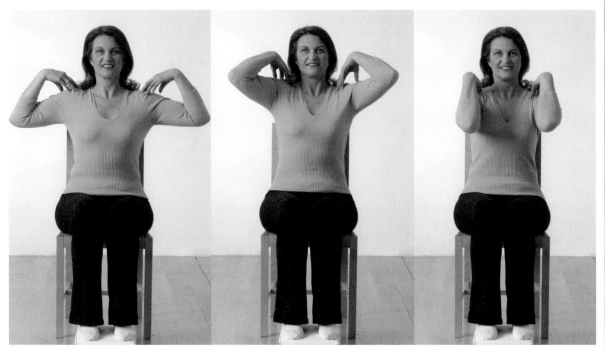

1 Sit up straight on a chair and place your hands on your shoulders so that your elbows stick out to the sides.

2 Very gently, draw circles in the air with your elbows, trying to imagine that you are oiling the inside of the joint.

3 Keep your circles small and stop if either shoulder feels strained. Circle forward five times and backward five times.

Sliding thumb

Sit up straight and try to slide your right thumb up your back, between your shoulder blades. See how high you can get. Now try with your left thumb. Does it go any higher? Note which side is stiffer.

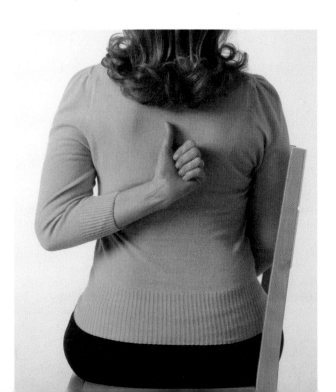

Frozen shoulder

Sitting deltoids

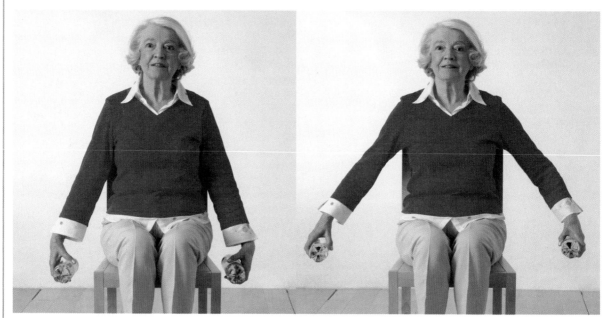

1 Hold a small bottle of water or a tin can in each hand. Alternatively, you can use weights if you have any, but not more than 400g weights in each hand. Sit up straight in a chair with your shoulders relaxed and your arms hanging by your sides. Breathe in.

2 Breathe out and engage your abdominals. Raise your arms out to the sides and, if you can, almost up to the level of your shoulders. Keep your shoulders down – don't let them hunch up as you lift your arms. Breathe in to lower your arms, and repeat five times.

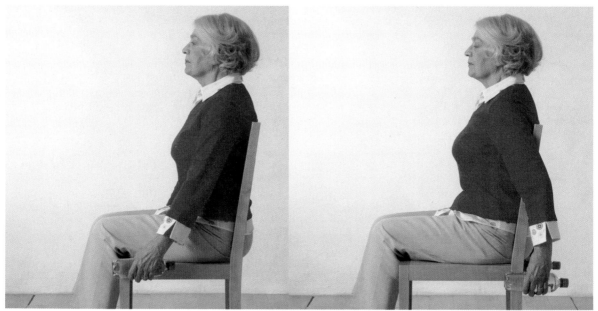

3 Repeat steps 1 and 2, but with your arms held roughly 10cm (4in) forward from the shoulder line.

4 Repeat steps 1 and 2, but with your arms held roughly 10cm (4in) back from the shoulder line.

The Windmill

1 Lie on your back with your knees bent. Place a folded towel under your head and another between your knees. Extend both arms straight up above your chest, palms facing forward and fingertips pointing to the ceiling. Breathe in.

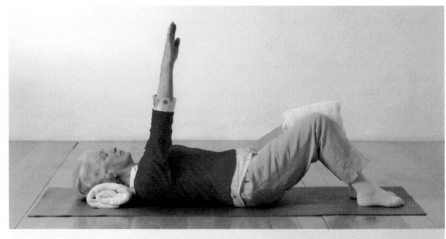

2 As you breathe out, engage your abdominals and lower your right arm to the floor by your hip. Lower your left arm to the floor by your left ear. Make sure that your back doesn't arch, and that the arm behind your head remains straight; if it starts to bend at the elbow and wrist, reduce the range of movement.

3 Breathe in to bring both arms back up to the centre, then breathe out to take your left arm down beside your hip and your right arm back by your head.

Repeat the sequence 10 times, alternating your arms and keeping a regular breathing pattern.

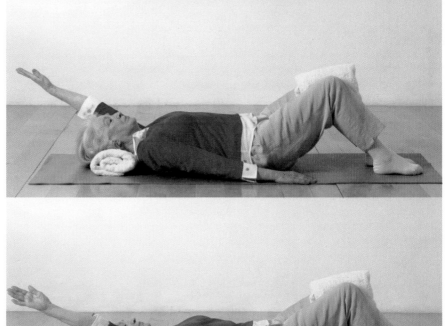

CAUTION: In other Pilates books, or in classes, you may come across a version of the Windmill in which you circle your arms above your head and in semi-circles down the sides. Don't attempt this if you have a shoulder problem.

Neck and upper back problems

Most commonly, problems in the upper back are the result of poor postural habits that may have developed over a number of years. The way you sit at a desk, at the dinner table, watch television, or drive the car can cause the shoulder muscles to bunch up until they feel hard, as if there are rocks inside them. Tight shoulder muscles make it difficult to twist round and look to the left or the right because you lose rotational flexibility. Perpetually hunched-up shoulders can also lead to knock-on problems in the neck, causing dizziness, nausea, shortness of breath, and even trapped nerves down one or both arms.

Kyphosis is an exaggerated forward curving of the upper spine, creating a humped appearance. There are several possible causes: it can be an inherited condition; it can be caused by diseases such as osteoporosis; and it can also develop as a result of years of poor posture. You can see early kyphosis in children who have a tendency to stoop, perhaps because they are shy or they're taller than other children in their class.

The forward curve of the upper back means that the head has to be lifted and the chin juts forward so that you can see straight ahead. This causes tension in the neck muscles. Also, because the weight of the upper body is leaning forward, the lower back has to take some of the strain in order for you to keep your balance.

Pilates can help to relieve the pain associated with kyphosis and upper back tension by strengthening the upper and middle back muscles. There's a huge, diamond-shaped muscle called the trapezius that stretches over this area, from the neck to the bottom of the shoulder blades, and it will often be bunched upward in those people who have upper back problems. Pilates exercises can lengthen these muscles, which in turn relieves the tension in the neck and shoulders.

CAUTION: If you have kyphosis, you should do as many different exercises as you can, but when lying on your back you should support your head and shoulders with pillows rather than trying to force that area down onto the floor. If you are receiving treatment for a neck problem, your specialist will advise you whether you need to mobilize or stabilize your neck; show him or her the exercises in this book before you try them. It may help if you support your head on a pillow or folded towel when doing exercises that involve your lying on your back. Be sure to avoid using shoulder bags, and follow the advice given on page 37 if you need to carry anything heavy.

Sitting lats with belt

The first course of action when trying to ease problems in the upper back and neck is to take work away from this area and focus on strengthening the mid back. You can do a straightforward version of Sitting lats (see p.63), or this version, which encourages rotational flexibility of the upper spine. Start with some Shoulder shrugs (p.62) to loosen your shoulders.

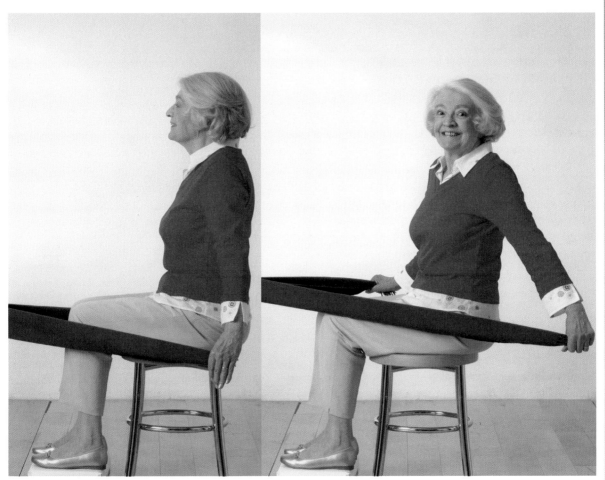

1 You'll need an elastic belt, or a scarf or an old pair of tights, plus a banister or door handle to loop it around. Sit on a stool with your thighs parallel to the floor. If necessary, place a book or yoga block under your feet. Hold the ends of the belt in each hand. Adjust the belt until it pulls tight when your arms are by your sides. Relax your shoulders, look ahead, and breathe in.

2 As you breathe out, engage your abdominals, slide your shoulder blades down, and pull the belt back with your left hand so that the right hand moves forward naturally. Try to feel the muscles working just at the base of your shoulder blade. Breathe in.

Breathe out and pull the belt back with your right hand so that the left hand moves forward naturally. Repeat five times in each direction.

Neck and upper back problems

Pillow squeeze

The serratus anterior muscle helps to pull the shoulder blades away from the spine toward your ribs. You can feel it working if you place your left hand on your ribs, just below the right armpit, then squeeze your right arm inward. This exercise works to strengthen the serratus anterior muscle.

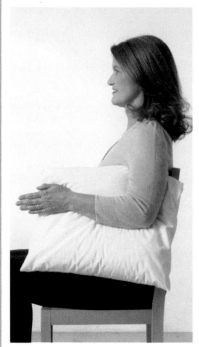

Sit up straight on a chair with your thighs parallel to the floor. Bend your left arm and place a folded pillow between your ribs and elbow. Relax your shoulders and breathe in. As you breathe out, squeeze the pillow for a count of five. Don't try to squeeze too hard – you should be able to feel the muscle pulling gently on your shoulder blade.

Repeat 10 times on each side.

Upper spine stretch

This stretch involves twisting your torso round to one side, and then to the other, while keeping your spine straight throughout.

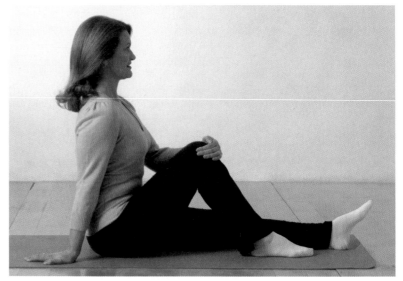

Sit up as straight as possible on the floor with both legs extended. Bend your right leg and rest your foot on the floor by your left calf. Place your right hand on the floor behind your right hip. Place your left hand across your right knee and look straight ahead.

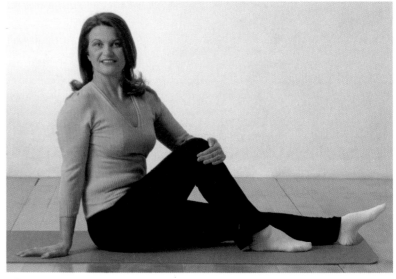

2 As you breathe out, engage your abdominals, lengthen your spine, and turn your torso to the right. Let your head follow the movement. Relax the spine as you breathe in, then breathe out on the right side again.

Repeat five times on each side.

Figure of eight

The main strategy for easing neck problems should be to correct your posture so that you hold your head correctly. However, there are a few exercises that can help to ease tension in the neck muscles themselves. This is one of them.

CAUTION: Don't try the Figure of eight or the neck stretches on page 84 if your doctor has told you to stabilize your neck.

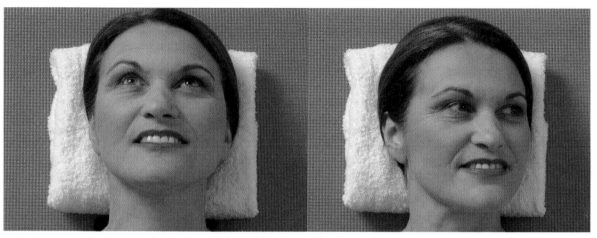

1 Lie on your back on the floor with your knees bent and your arms by your sides. Place a folded towel under your head so that your spine is straight. Imagine that there is a blackboard just above your face, and a piece of chalk on the tip of your nose. You are going to write the figure "8" on the blackboard with your nose. Breathe in.

2 As you breathe out, lightly engage your abdominals and very slowly draw the first loop to one side. You'll have to lift slightly to reach the outside of the loop.

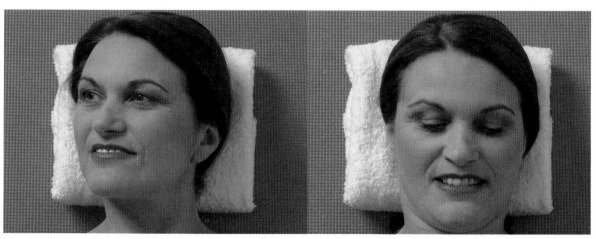

3 Continue the motion by drawing the second loop on the other side with your nose.

4 Finish your first 8, then breathe in. Breathe out and begin another figure 8, making your movements slow.

Repeat five times on each side.

Neck and upper back problems

Neck stretches

This exercise lengthens the muscles in the back of the neck.

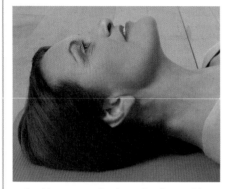

| Lie on your back on the floor with your arms by your sides. Don't use a support under your head. Breathe in and slowly lift your chin right up.

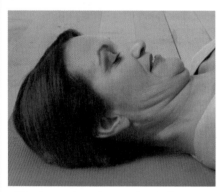

2 As you breathe out, slowly drop your chin right down. Keep the rest of your body relaxed.

Repeat several times.

Isometric neck exercises

These exercises can be very helpful for people who have lost muscle strength in their neck and find it difficult to hold their head straight. They can be done even if your doctor has told you to stabilize your neck.

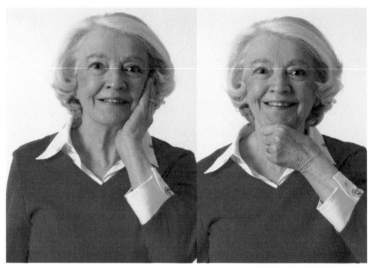

| Sit in front of a mirror with your back straight and your feet on the floor. Shrug your shoulders and let them fall naturally into place. Place your left palm against the left side of your face and press gently against it without letting your head move. Hold for five seconds. You should feel the muscles on the left side of your neck working to resist the pressure. Check in the mirror that you're not letting your head move.

Repeat the action on the right side.

2 Make a loose fist and press it up against your chin without moving your head. The muscles at the front of your neck should be working to resist the push of your fist.

3 Make a loose fist and press it against your forehead. This time you'll feel the muscles in front of your ears working.

Repeat all these movements four times, holding each for five seconds.

Breathing problems

There can be many reasons why people find they get out of breath more easily as they get older. Perhaps they have damaged their lungs from years of smoking, or maybe they have a lung disorder of some kind. In many cases, it is a combination of poor posture and failure to use the entire lung capacity on a regular basis, so they've lost the habit of breathing correctly.

Chronic obstructive lung disease is a blanket term encompassing a range of chest disorders, including asthma, emphysema, and chronic bronchitis. In all of these cases, the respiratory system isn't working efficiently so the sufferer may experience coughing, wheezing, and short-ness of breath from even mild exertion. This may make you reluctant to exercise, but in fact increased muscle strength will help you to breathe more easily if you choose the right activity.

Pilates is an especially good choice because if you correct your posture and strengthen the upper body muscles, the lungs are able to work with less effort. Pilates teaches a slow, steady breathing pattern and, since it does not aim to increase the heart rate, you shouldn't find it too strenuous. Practise all the upper body exercises in the previous section, and do the breathing ones in this section as well.

CAUTION: Don't take any risks if you have chronic obstructive lung disease. Work under the supervision of a qualified teacher until you are confident that you can manage on your own.

Semi-supine breathing

You can do this breathing practice while sitting or standing, as well as lying down. Keep practising it whenever you have a moment to spare during the day, and you'll find that your breathing muscles will soon get stronger.

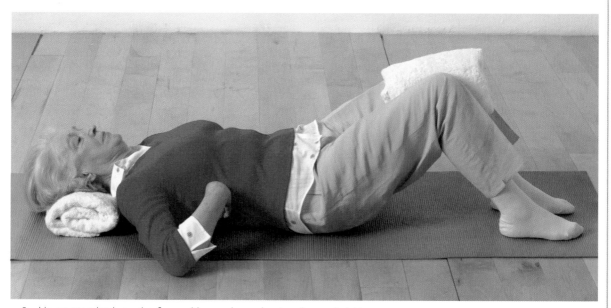

Lie on your back on the floor with your knees bent and your feet hip-width apart. Support your head with a folded towel. Place the backs of your hands on your ribs, just below your armpits. Breathe in through your nose and feel your ribs pushing your hands outward.

Breathe out through your mouth and feel your ribs move in again.

Breathing problems

Side-lying breathing

This exercise is particularly beneficial if you suffer from scoliosis, since it helps you to concentrate your breathing on one side of your lungs at a time.

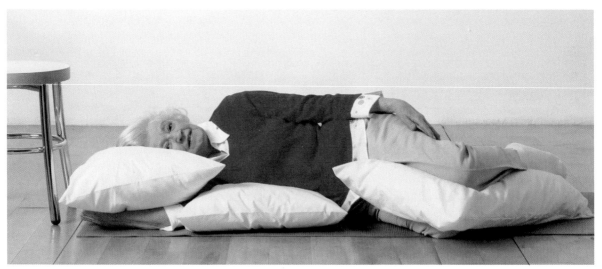

1 Position a low stool next to you, then lie on your right side on the floor and extend your right arm along the floor. Place one pillow under your ribs and another between your head and your right arm.

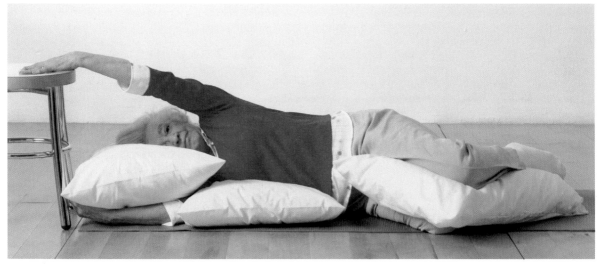

2 Stretch your left arm up over your head so that your left hand touches the seat of the stool. Breathe into your left side. Breathe out and release your left arm back down.

Repeat on each side four times.

Lower back pain

There can be several causes of lower back pain, but almost invariably the condition will be accompanied by weak abdominal muscles. The way to fix this is to strengthen the abdominals. Stomach muscles can be weak for various reasons: if you are overweight, you have never regained muscle tone after a pregnancy, you have had abdominal surgery, or you simply haven't exercised them enough.

When your abdominals don't support your spine, you become prone to a condition called lordosis, which is an excessive curvature of the lower spine. Your bottom sticks out at the back and your stomach hangs out at the front. Wearing high heels can also be a factor in causing this condition, since the shoes tilt the pelvis forward, forcing you to lean back to keep your balance and thus emphasizing the lower back curve. The muscles in the lower back and hip area shorten and the pelvis moves out of its correct alignment, leading to lower back pain in the short term and all sorts of problems in the long term. Such problems could include disc prolapse or walking difficulties.

Pilates can help to correct all these problems by strengthening the stomach, glute, hamstring, and pelvic floor muscles, and thus correcting the pelvic alignment.

CAUTION: When lying on your back, it may help if you put your feet up on a stool or pad. This will enable you to lower your back to the floor without straining it. Lordosis sufferers should also be particularly careful when lifting or carrying because they could easily strain their back (see pp.36–37 for advice on this subject).

Are You Overweight?

The simplest way to assess whether you need to reduce your weight is to calculate your body mass index (BMI). To do this, you divide your weight in kilograms by the square of your height in metres:

weight ÷ [height x height] = BMI

Check your score:

Less than 15	**Emaciated**
15–19	**Underweight**
19–25	**Fine**
25–30	**Overweight**
Over 30	**Obese**

If your BMI is over 25 or under 19, contact your doctor for advice. If you are underweight, you are at risk of nutritional deficiencies, which can lead to fractures and other health problems. If you are overweight, you will be putting a lot of strain on your lower back, hips, knees, and feet, and you are likely to develop bad posture if your stomach muscles aren't strong enough to keep your spine and pelvis in correct alignment.

Carrying too much weight can cause all kinds of health problems, no matter what age you are. If you are on a weight-loss diet, focus on strengthening your stomach muscles for the first few weeks. Pilates can help to tone up flabby areas very quickly and you'll be more motivated when you see the results of your efforts.

Ab curls

The ab curls you do in Pilates have little to do with the sit-ups you may have learned in an aerobics class, although the movements may look the same. The Pilates ab curl uses the three major muscle groups of the abdomen: transverse abdominals, which run across the abdomen and hold all the organs in place; the obliques at your sides, which help the body to rotate; and the rectus abdominus down the front, which enables the body to bend forward. Standard sit-ups just use the rectus abdominus and they can easily strain the neck and lower back.

The Pilates ab curl is a very slow, careful movement, and it's important to concentrate on getting the right sensations to make sure that you are using your muscles correctly.

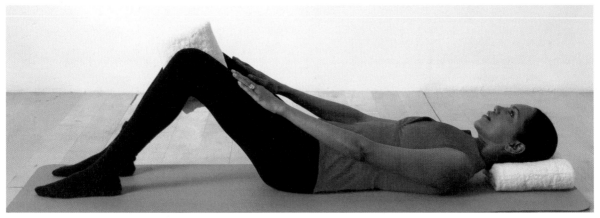

1 Lie on your back with your knees bent. Place a folded towel between your knees and another under your head. Rest your hands on your thighs. If you have trouble keeping your back flat, rest your lower legs on a chair. Relax your shoulders and breathe in.

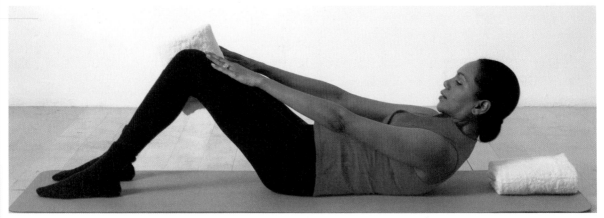

2 As you breathe out, pull your abdominals toward the floor. Slide your hands up toward your knees and move your shoulder blades slightly down your back as you lift your upper torso and head off the floor. Curl your ribs forward in the direction of your thighs, but don't feel you have to lift very far; a small lift is fine because you'll get most of the benefit from the first few centimetres of movement.

CAUTION: Did you feel any strain in your lower back? Be sure that you don't start to curl until you can feel that your abdominals are engaged. Keep your neck soft and curl up from the abdomen; don't pull up with your head and shoulders.

Breathe in to curl back down again. Repeat 10 times.

Cross-fibre ab curls

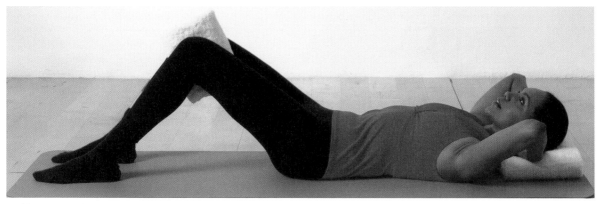

1 Lie on your back with your knees bent. Place a folded towel between your knees, and another under your head. Place both hands behind your head and breathe in.

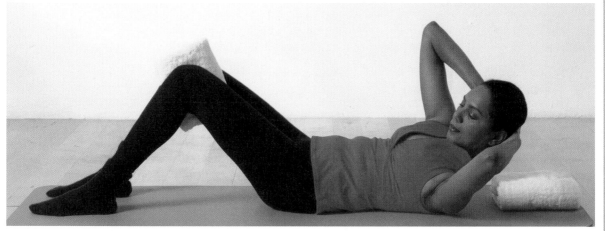

2 As you breathe out, engage your abdominals and lift your right shoulder off the floor. Draw your right elbow toward the your left hip.

Pause, then breathe in as you curl back down again. Repeat 10 times on each side.

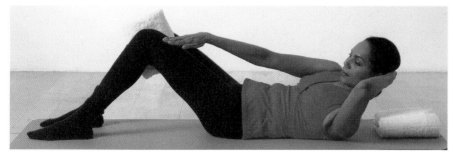

Variation
As you breathe out, engage your abdominals and curl your right shoulder towards your left hip, stretching your right hand past your left knee.

CAUTION: You shouldn't feel any strain in your neck as you curl upwards. If you do, try placing a small folded towel under your upper back and head and hold the corners between your fingers. As you curl forward, pull the towel so that it supports your head.

Ab curls

Reverse curl

If you are having trouble with the ab curls described on the previous pages, try this alternative method of strengthening your abdominals instead.

1 Sit up straight on the floor with your knees bent and your arms straight out in front of you. Breathe in.

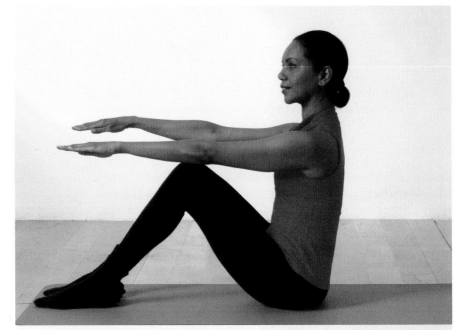

2 As you breathe out, engage your abdominals and roll your back down toward the floor, using your stomach muscles to control the curl. Don't try to go all the way down; your muscles will be working most effectively when you are at an angle of roughly 45 degrees.

Breathe in and use your hands to help you lift your torso upright again. Keep your back straight at all times. Repeat five times.

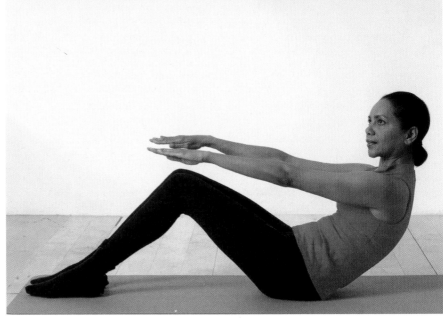

Double leg lift

Don't try this exercise until your abdominals are already quite strong, and stop immediately if you feel any twinges in your lower back.

CAUTION: Don't let your legs swing back as you lift; keep them in line with the pelvis. If you find this tricky, move your legs forward slightly and lift from that angle until your muscles are stronger.

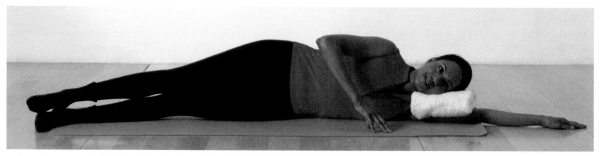

1 Lie on your left side with your legs straight, one above the other. Check that your shoulders are directly above each other too, and that your hip bones are in line. If necessary, place a cushion under your waist to prevent it sinking into the floor. Extend your lower arm under your head and insert a rolled-up towel to support your head. Rest the fingers of your right hand lightly on the floor in front of you. When you are ready, breathe in.

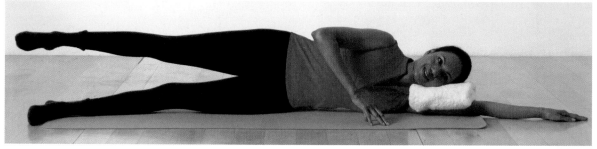

2 As you breathe out, engage your abdominals and stretch both legs down through the heels before you raise the right leg off the ground. Only lift up a few centimetres, then breathe in and release down. Do five repetitions on each side.

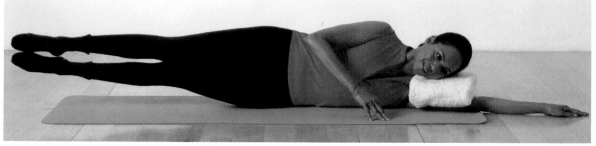

3 Next, as you breathe out, engage your abdominals and try lifting both legs off the ground. Breathe in, and release down. Do five repetitions on each side. When you lift both legs, it might help if you place a pillow between the thighs so that you remember to squeeze them together.

More exercises for lower back pain

After working the abdominals in a Pilates session, you should turn over to lie on your front and do some Glute squeezes (see p.58) and then some Hamstring curls (see p.59). Turn onto your back and finish up with the back stretch you did in bed (see pp.26–27), moving your knees slowly round an imaginary clock face.

After any abdominal surgery, check with your doctor before starting gentle abdominal exercises. Begin by pulling in your abs while sitting in a chair or in the car. Next, try Side-lying static abs (see pp.22–23). When you have enough muscle strength to do these confidently, move on to Ab curls and Cross-fibre ab curls (see pp.90–91).

Pelvic floor

The pelvic floor muscles run in a kind of hammock between your legs, and help to control the openings of the urethra, vagina (in women), and anus. If they weaken, they can cause incontinence (both urinary and bowel), and women risk prolapse of the uterus. Strengthening them has many benefits, not least for your sex life.

You can engage your pelvic floor muscles in exercises such as Pelvic tilts (see p.51) to help move your pelvis. You will also find it helpful to engage your pelvic muscles while doing Glute squeezes and Hamstring curls. To work the pelvic floor effectively, you need to isolate different areas of the muscles.

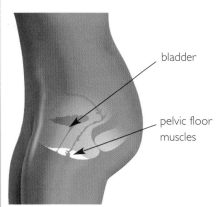

bladder

pelvic floor muscles

The pelvic floor muscles help to hold your pelvis in correct alignment.

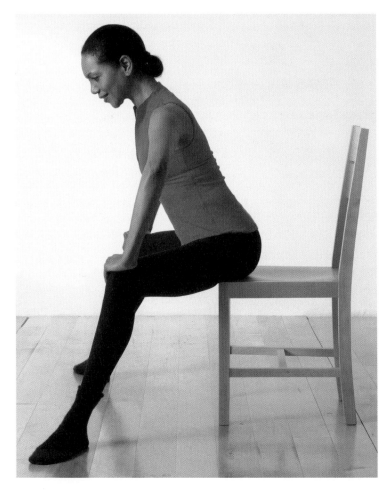

Sit on a chair with your knees as far apart as you can manage and with your feet flat on the floor. Lean forward from the waist and place your hands on your knees to support your back and keep it straight. Keep your shoulder blades down. Imagine that you are pulling your bladder toward your rib cage. Feel the internal lift of this movement.

Hold for five seconds, then release. Repeat 10 times.

Scoliosis

Scoliosis is when the spine curves to one side. Sometimes it may cause the spine to curve to one side at the top, and to the opposite side in the lower spine, causing an "S" shape. Scoliosis frequently starts in childhood while the bones are still developing, either as a result of a fall or bump on the tailbone, or from a habit such as carrying a heavy school bag on one side of the body, day in, day out. Knock-knees, rolling the weight onto the inside of the foot, or uneven leg lengths can also cause scoliosis unless they are corrected, as your body adjusts to cope with the misalignment in the pelvis. There are different degrees of scoliosis, and the treatments for the most severe cases can include surgery to insert a rod in the spine, or wearing corsets or braces. You should always gets expert medical advice about scoliosis: if left untreated, it will get worse.

Pilates can help in most cases if you work to strengthen the weaker side, and create strong abdominal and pelvic muscles to help the spine to straighten. Get an instructor to work out an individual programme that suits your body.

CAUTION: Follow your specialist's advice on which moves or exercises to avoid. You will probably be told to avoid anything that causes trauma to the pelvic area, such as horse-riding or, heaven forbid, bungee jumping!

Uneven leg lengths

This is quite common, especially among young people, and you can see why it may lead to scoliosis if left untreated: there is a tendency to lean into the shorter leg, forcing the spine to curve in order to keep the centre of gravity down the middle of the body.

If your leg length discrepancy is less than a centimetre, you may be able to compensate for this by strengthening the muscles that support the pelvis. If it's more than a centimetre, you should see a specialist who will probably recommend that you wear shoes with a heel lift on the shorter side.

CAUTION: The important thing to remember with uneven leg lengths is to avoid leaning into the shorter leg, habitually sitting with your weight balanced into one hip, or crossing your legs. If you do any of these, the muscles on one side will shorten over time, and the condition will be much harder to correct.

Sciatica

When the posture in the lower spine is poor, the sciatic nerve that runs from the pelvis through the buttocks and thighs can become trapped, causing pain and numbness in the area. It's important to get a medical diagnosis, since different things can cause the pressure on the nerve, and there will be separate treatments for each. However, you can help to ease it by correcting your posture throughout daily life: never slump into your lower back when sitting, and be very careful when lifting.

Pilates exercises that strengthen the core posture muscles can help (Ab curls, Pelvic tilts, Glute squeezes, Hamstring curls), but check with your specialist about which are safe for you, as you could inflame the problem if you're not careful.

Hip replacements

A hip replacement operation will usually be recommended when the cartilage in the hip joint has worn down so much that the ball at the top of the thigh bone and the socket in the pelvic bone grind against each other. Little bony growths, known as osteocytes, may form in the area. Hip replacement is now an enormously successful operation and the new generation of implants can last a lifetime, whereas a couple of decades ago they may have lasted 10 to15 years.

Before surgery, it is important to strengthen the muscles of the pelvis, thighs, stomach, and bottom as much as possible because this will help the area to heal more quickly. After surgery, follow your specialist's advice for the first few months, and thereafter you can return to exercising as normal, with a few precautions.

**Exercises to strengthen muscles
before an operation:**
Practise Glute squeezes (see p.58), Hamstring curls (see p.59), Outer thigh lifts (see p.57) and Inner thigh – sitting (see p.68). Work within a range of movement that feels comfortable and stop if you feel any pain.

Exercises to try after an operation:
You will have to learn to balance your weight across both legs correctly, since before the operation you leant your weight into the good side. Once you are standing and walking again, engage your abdominals and squeeze your glutes slightly to get the correct pelvic alignment, and try to keep your hip bones level. At first you will be told to climb stairs one by one, leading with the "good" side on the way up and the "bad" side on the way down. Once your specialist gives the all-clear, you can practise properly balanced stair-climbing and descending (see pp.34–35).

Do all the exercises recommended for before the operation, plus as many as you like from the Top-to-toe workout, but don't ever take your leg across the centre line of the body.

Weak at the knees

Knees are particularly prone to arthritis, as the discs of joint cartilage wear down over time. You can protect them to an extent by keeping the muscles that support the knee joint strong, and avoiding bending the knee when it is not correctly aligned. Sports that involve running and turning suddenly, such as football, rugby, and basketball, can damage the ligaments that hold the knee joint in position. Habitually sitting with your legs crossed also weakens the ligaments.

Knee replacements are used when the cartilage has worn down to such an extent that there is extreme pain and limited or no mobility. Before and after surgery, it is important to strengthen the quadricep muscles at the front of the thighs, and the hamstrings at the back, since they are the main muscles for bending and straightening the knee joints. It is important that these muscles are strengthened equally to allow the knees to work in good alignment. In Pilates you are also taught to straighten your posture so that the pelvis is correctly aligned and not putting undue strain on one knee or the other.

Within a couple of months of a knee replacement operation, you will be able to bear your full weight on the knee, but you should make sure that it tracks correctly at all times (with the kneecap pointing forward).

CAUTION: Avoid any movements that twist the knee – football and skiing are not a good idea. Don't ever kneel with your lower legs splayed out to the sides. Keep your knees slightly "soft" when you are exercising and don't "lock" them. If you injure a knee ligament, take the advice of a specialist before exercising again.

Exercises to support the knee joint

If you have weak knees, you should start working on the back of the leg first, doing some Glute squeezes (see p.58) and Hamstring curls (see p.59) at the start of every exercise session. The calf exercises that you do lying in bed, pointing and flexing your feet (see p.29), are also very good, and the exercises on pages 98–100 are all designed to strengthen the muscles that support the knee joint.

Inner thighs – lying

This is slightly trickier than the Inner thigh – sitting exercise (see p.68). If you have any trouble, do the sitting version until your inner thigh muscles are stronger.

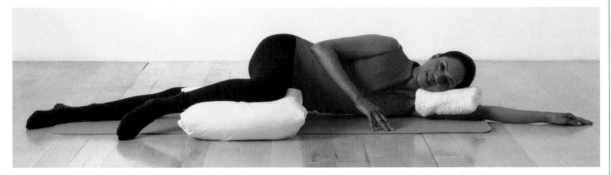

1 Lie on your left side on the floor and extend your arm. Place a folded towel under your head. Bend your right leg 90 degrees and rest the knee on a pillow. Slightly bend the bottom leg so that your heel is in line with your tailbone. Check that your shoulder joints and your hip bones are in line and that your spine is straight. Breathe in.

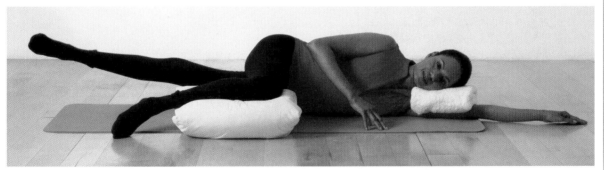

2 Breathe out, engage your abdominals, stretch the right leg out through the heel, and gently lift it off the floor. Lift as high as you can, but make sure that there is no movement in the rest of your body.

Hold for five seconds, then breathe in as you lower your leg again. Repeat five times on each side, making sure that your spine stays straight and your shoulders and hips don't roll forward.

Weak at the knees

Strengthening the quads

This exercise works the quadriceps at the fronts of the thighs, as well as the calf and ankle muscles.

1 Arrange a pile of pillows so that you can lie on your back with your right leg resting over the pillows and your left leg bent, with the left foot resting on the floor by the side of the pillows. Breathe in.

2 As you breathe out, engage your abdominals and extend your right leg until it is straight. Flex the foot.

3 Breathe in and hold your stomach muscles, then point your right foot.

4 Breathe out, keeping your abdominals engaged, and flex your right foot again.

5 Breathe in and lower your flexed foot down to the floor.

Repeat five times with each leg.

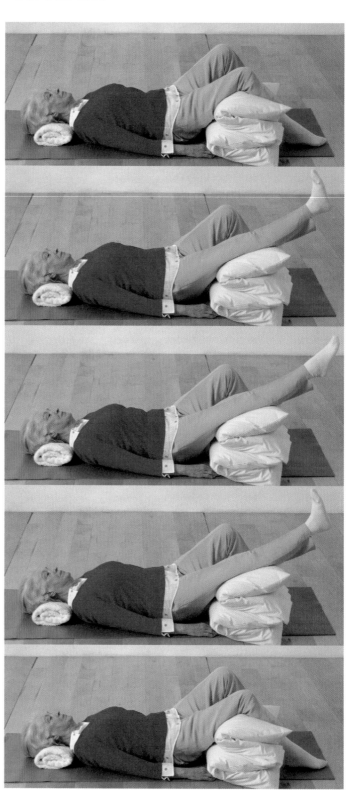

Back of
the knee stretch

Always follow a quads
exercise with a back
of the knee stretch.
You can also do this
after cycling or running,
or any other form of
activity that works the
front of the thighs.

1 Sit on the floor with
one leg extended and
a folded towel under
the knee. The other leg
should be bent with the
foot resting on the floor.
Support your upright
position by keeping your
hands on the floor behind
you. Make sure that your
back is straight. Breathe in.

2 As you breathe
out, engage your
abdominals, lean
forward from the hips, and
gently press your knee
down into the towel. Put
your right hand on your left
knee. Flex your foot and
feel the stretch in the back
of your knee.

Sit up again and repeat on
the other side.

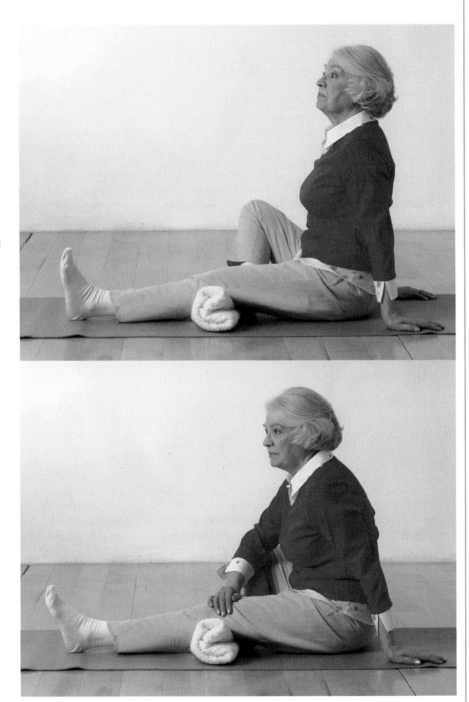

Weak at the knees

Hamstring stretch

Do a hamstring stretch any time the backs of your legs feel tight, and in every exercise session that focuses on legs.

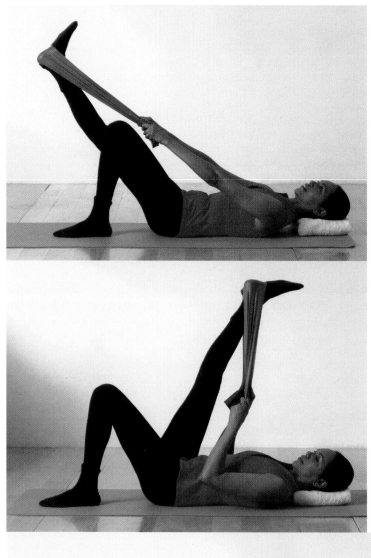

1 Lie on your back facing a wall, so that you can place your right heel against the wall if necessary. Bend the left knee. Loop an elasticated belt or towel around the right foot and hold the ends in your hands. As you breathe in, engage your abdominals, press into your heel and hold the stretch for a few seconds.

2 Breathe out slowly, drawing your leg towards your chest by pulling the ends of the belt. You'll feel the stretch in the back of your leg. Pull as far as you can manage, then lower your leg to the floor.

Repeat four times each side.

3 Try the same exercise again, but this time place both ends of the belt in your right hand. Pull your left leg across your body towards the right shoulder, and vice versa for the right leg.

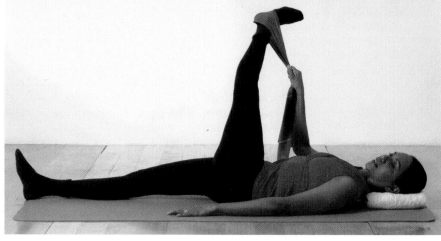

Feet and ankle problems

Most exercise programmes ignore feet, but painful foot and ankle conditions can be severely debilitating for older people, and can lead to a total loss of mobility. If your feet are sore, you won't balance your weight squarely through them, your ankles will be forced to one side or the other, your knees won't track properly, and strain will be put on the hip joints and thus on the spine.

Check an old pair of shoes to see where they wore down first. If the heels are worn down while the soles are more or less intact, you are leaning your weight backward. You may find that your toes bend up to help you keep your balance when standing. Conversely, if the soles are more worn than the heels, you're leaning forward and your toes may bend under like claws to support you. Are your shoes more worn on the insides or the outsides? Rolling your feet inward causes knock-kneed postures, while rolling them out gives a bow-legged appearance.

Bunions, flat feet, and any other foot problems will affect the way you balance your weight and thus the alignment of the rest of your body. Lack of mobility in the ankle joint can severely restrict walking because your foot is not able to move up and down freely. Pilates can't fix damage that has already been done, but it can help you to strengthen your feet and ankle muscles to enable them to work more effectively.

CAUTION: Don't wear silly shoes! Very high heels force the entire body into an unnatural posture and should never be worn for long periods. A lowish heel is fine, so long as the heel of the shoe is positioned directly underneath the front of your heel – not the back – so that your weight is transmitted straight downward. Shoes that don't hold your instep firmly – either they are too loose or cut too low over the arch – will cause you to tense your muscles in an effort to keep them on. And shoes that pinch in one area cause you to shift your weight from the site of the pain.

Foot massage

Do this for yourself or see if you can get someone else to do it for you. It's particularly good if you are prone to cramp in the feet.

1 Stroke the whole foot firmly from heel to toes to encourage circulation. It can help if you use a massage oil, or some baby oil.

2 Apply firmer pressure to the base of each toe with your thumbs, stretching the joints away from the rest of the foot.

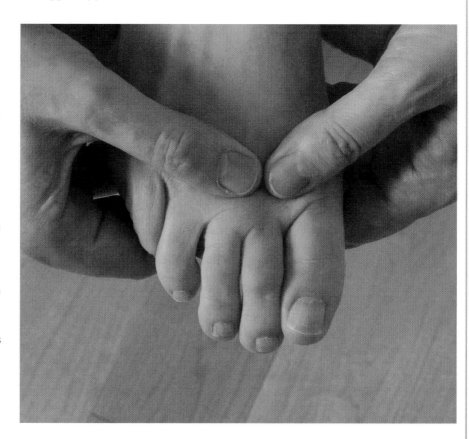

Feet and ankle problems

Doming the feet

Do this exercise at any time of day, but always with bare feet so that
you can move the muscles in each foot more easily.

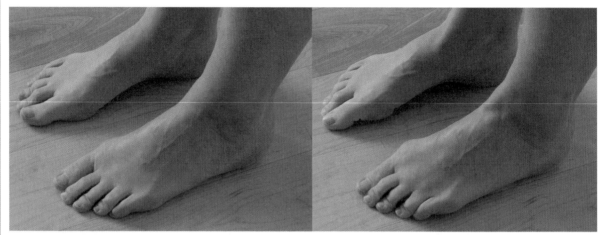

1 Sit up straight on a chair with your feet firmly planted
on the floor. Make sure that your weight is evenly
distributed between the heel and both sides of the
front of the foot, in a kind of triangle shape.

2 Keeping your heels on the floor, draw the toes on
one foot back so that your instep is raised. Don't let
the toes curl under.

Hold for a few seconds then return to the starting position.

Repeat 10 times with each foot.

Heel and toe

Try this exercise whenever you have the opportunity while sitting in a chair.
You can exercise each foot separately or together.

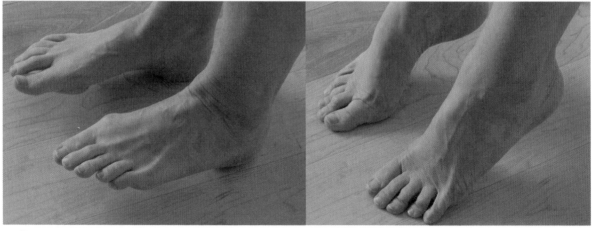

1 Sit up straight on the chair with your feet flat on the
floor. Lift all your toes off the floor, as high as you
possibly can.

2 Lower the toes and lift your heels up high.
Repeat the action 10 times.

Calf raises

Keep this movement very slow and controlled, and always make sure that you are leaning against something for support.

| Stand up straight with your hands resting on the back of a chair. Keep your feet flat on the floor. Breathe in.

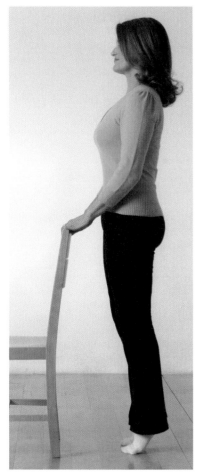

2 As you breathe out, engage your abdominals, squeeze your glutes, and slowly lift up onto the balls of your feet.

Hold for five seconds, then roll down again. Repeat 10 times.

Calf strengthening

This works the muscles on the outsides of the calves, which help to prevent the feet rolling inward or outward.

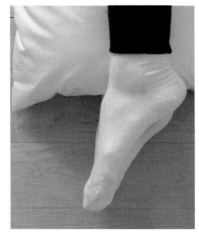

| Lie on your side with your back against a wall and both legs straight. Place a pillow between your lower legs. Breathe in.

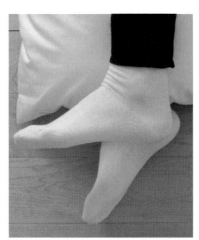

2 As you breathe out, point and flex the top foot, feeling the stretch in the side of your calf.

Repeat five times with each foot.

Calf stretches

| Stand up straight with your hands resting on the back of a chair and a yoga block or a book on the floor in front of you. Rest the ball of your left foot against the edge of the block or book so that your foot is curled upward. Your heel should remain on the floor.

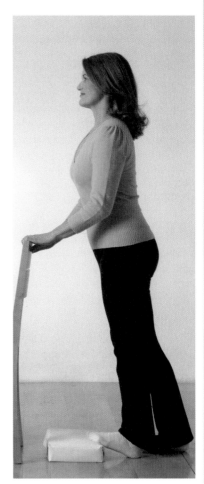

2 Lean forward, keeping your back straight, and you'll feel a stretch in your calf.

Hold for a few seconds, then repeat on the other side.

Heart disease

If you have angina, coronary heart disease, or you have had heart surgery, the thought of exercise can be terrifying, but it's important for you to do as much as you can. Your specialist should give you an exercise ECG (electrocardiogram) in which your heart activity is recorded while you cycle on an exercise bike or walk on a treadmill. This will help the doctors to diagnose the severity of your condition and determine the level of exercise that is safe for you.

The normal recommendation is that you do half an hour of aerobic activity – that is, working the heart and lungs – at least five days a week. You can start with brisk walking, then gradually

Exercises to help the circulation

Try doing as many exercises as you can from the Top-to-toe workout, but keep your legs elevated whenever you have the option. When the instruction is to lie in the semi-supine position on your back with your knees bent, lie with your feet up on a chair. You could buy a physio ball to support your legs as you work out. This piece of equipment is widely available to buy by mail order or from stores with a fitness section. You can use a physio ball to do Ab curls or Hip rolls, for example, or practise sitting on one to improve your balance. A physio ball also helps to isolate the abdominal muscles by preventing you from pressing down through your thighs.

Feet and ankle point and flex

1 Lie on your back with your head resting on a folded towel. Bend your right leg and rest your foot on the floor. Relax your arms at your sides. Place your lower left leg on a physio ball if you have one, or on a stool. Flex the left foot so that your toes point toward the ceiling. Point and flex 10 times, then swap legs and repeat on the other side.

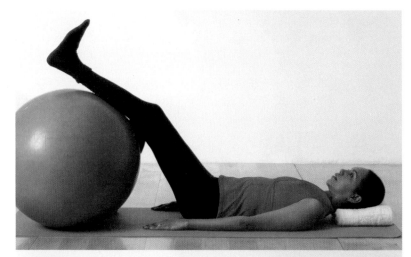

2 Point your toes away from you. Circle them in a clockwise and then anticlockwise direction.

Repeat with the other leg. When you are feeling stronger, place both feet on the ball to do this exercise.

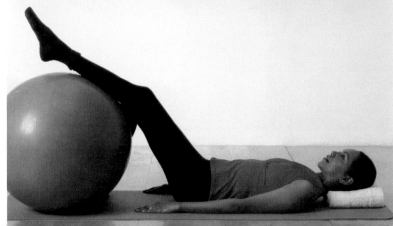

then gradually increase the distance covered, or switch to aerobic exercises such as swimming, cycling, tennis, or jogging, as you feel able.

Pilates is non-aerobic, but it can strengthen your muscles to make it easier for you to work aerobically. For example, if you suffer from blockages in the arteries in your legs, Pilates can stretch and tone the leg muscles safely. This will encourage the growth of new blood vessels, control pain, and increase the distance you walk.

CAUTION: Always stop if you get tired, short of breath, or suffer chest pains.

Kicking legs

1 Lie on your back, with your head resting on a folded towel, and your arms relaxed at your sides. Lift both feet off the floor and bend your knees.

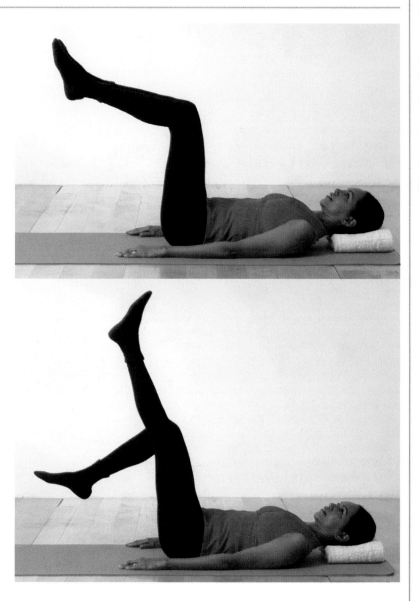

2 Breathe out, engage your abdominal muscles and raise one leg then the other so that your thighs are at right angles to the floor (or as close to this as possible) and your knees are together. Kick up your legs alternately – left leg up and right leg down, right leg up and left leg down – while breathing frequently. Repeat 10 times.

When you feel strong enough, curl your upper body forward to activate the abs more effectively as you lift each leg up.

Stroke recovery

Strokes occur when the blood flow to the brain is interrupted, and the damage they cause depends on the area of the brain they affect and their severity.

Immediately after a stroke, the medical team will assess the damage and advise on the rehabilitation and exercise that should be undertaken to enhance recovery. It's important to get the joints moving as soon as possible after a stroke under the guidance of a qualified professional. Pilates can be extremely effective in stroke recovery because of its focus on correct posture and strengthening both large and small muscle groups. Exercises that promote balance and co-ordination are helpful and, once there is sufficient strength and control, moderate aerobic exercise can be beneficial for the circulation.

CAUTION: Avoid rapid movements of the head and neck, or lowering the head below the level of the hips. Take care that any weak areas of the body are supported rather than hanging loose, which could induce swelling.

Osteoporosis

Osteoporosis is a gradual loss of bone density, primarily affecting the spine, hips, and wrists, and the risk of fractures at these sites is greatly increased. It is more common in women, particularly post-menopausal women, but men can get it too. The incidence of osteoporosis is rising rapidly in the 21st century, perhaps because we are leading increasingly sedentary lifestyles, but if you are diagnosed with the disease there is a lot you can do to help yourself.

In particular, it has been shown that a regular exercise programme can halt the progression of the disease. Pilates is ideal because it is low-impact and totally safe when done correctly. By strengthening all the muscles that support the spine and pelvis, and improving your posture so that force is applied correctly on the joints, you can also minimize your risk of fracture.

CAUTION: There are a number of movements you should avoid, both when exercising and in everyday life. Don't bend your spine forward, especially when lifting something; keep your back straight, and bend at the hips without twisting. Don't rotate your spine sideways, whether in a sitting or standing position.

Disability

If you are confined to a wheelchair, it is vital that you retain as much muscle tone as possible. Whether you have a manual or a powered chair, there is a tendency to hunch forward to operate it, which could cause shoulder and neck problems over time. You can counteract this by focusing on Pilates exercises that pull muscles in the opposite direction and strengthen the mid and upper back muscles. Strong stomach muscles also prevent you slumping into your lower back and risking potential problems in that area.

If you use a Zimmer frame or crutches to get around, you should first and foremost make sure that the equipment is adjusted to the correct height. Strengthening the stomach muscles can be very beneficial in helping you to retain a good posture while using your walking aids.

CAUTION: If you have a single crutch or walking stick, restrict the time you spend using it. Any activity in which you regularly lean your weight to one side will have repercussions on your joints and muscles before too long.

Exercises for wheelchair users

Whenever you remember, pull your stomach muscles back to keep them as strong as possible. To strengthen the upper and mid back, do Shoulder shrugs (see p.62), Sitting lats (see p.63), Working the upper torso (see pp.64–65), Pillow squeeze (see p.84), and Cossack Arms (see p.33). You can also try Side bends holding the opposite arm of the chair (see p.67).

Shoulder stretch

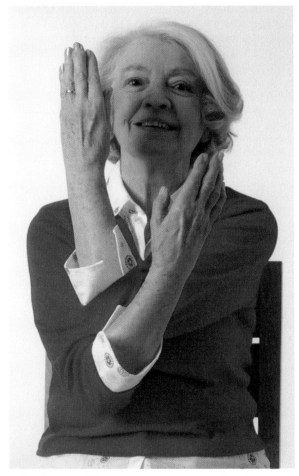

Sit up straight and cross your arms at the elbows so that both arms are in front of your chest. Breathe in. As you breathe out, engage your abdominals and draw your left arm across your body at the elbow using your right forearm.

Hold the stretch for five seconds, then repeat with the other arm.

Thoracic stretch

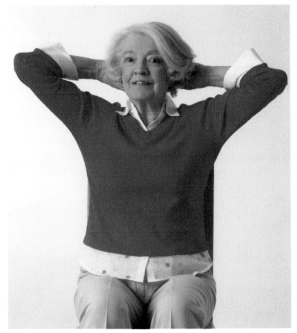

Sit up straight with both hands placed on the back of your neck. Slide your hands up to the top of your head.

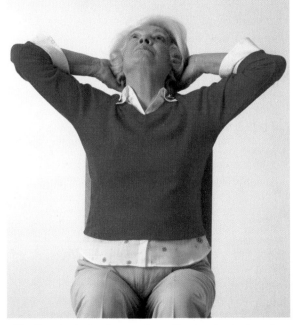

2 Breathe in. Look up at the ceiling, leaning back as far as possible. Hold for five seconds. Repeat a few times.

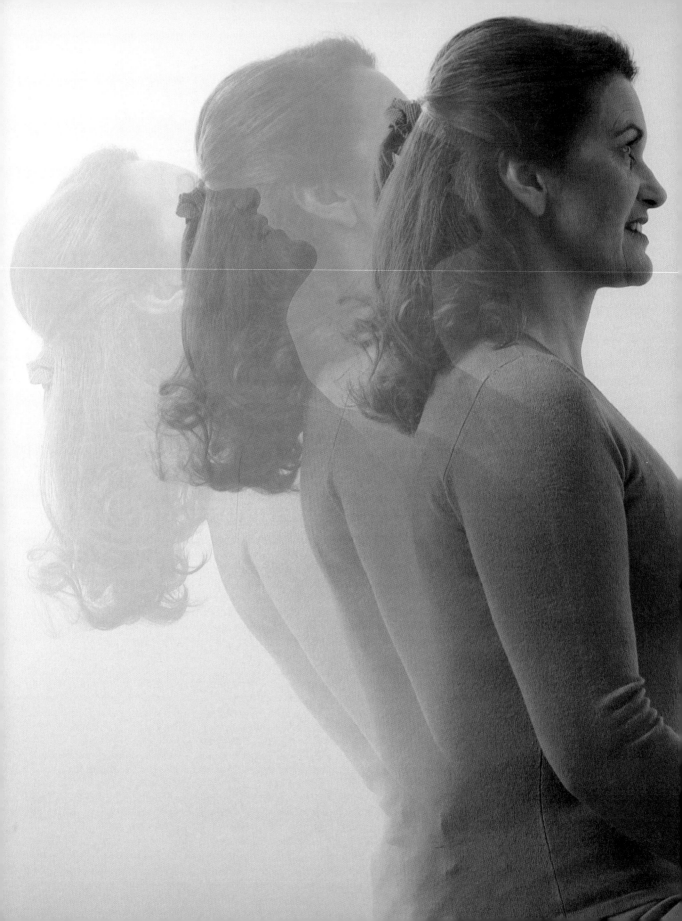

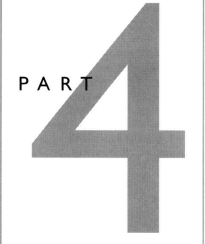

PART **4**

Creating change

Now that you have learned some basic exercises to help keep you in shape and remedy any imbalances, the next step is to keep doing them. At first, the benefits will be so obvious that they will provide motivation in themselves, but in the longer term it is important to chart your progress from time to time and reassess yourself against some benchmarks.

It could become boring doing exactly the same routine every time, so in this chapter you will find three more workouts of varying degrees of difficulty, plus some tips on how to create your own personal plan. Make Pilates an integral part of your lifestyle and you can look forward to a body that remains as flexible and mobile as it possibly can for the rest of your life.

Setting goals

You should aim to do at least two hours of Pilates and two hours of aerobic exercise every week. The Pilates exercises can either comprise two hour-long sessions in which you cover all the main muscle groups, or you can break it down into several shorter sessions at which you focus on just one area at a time (such as abdominals, lats, or legs). If you also maintain an awareness of Pilates in your daily activities, you can help to build muscle strength as you go about your everyday chores.

On pages 14 and 15 you learned how to assess your own posture and self-diagnose imbalances and asymmetrical areas. Try this again after a month of doing Pilates exercises on a regular basis and see if you can spot any differences. Are your shoulders and hips more even? Is your stomach flatter? Are you balancing your weight evenly through your feet? Which areas still need work? Repeat this reassessment every month or so, and adjust your exercise programme to focus on the areas that need to be strengthened.

You can also chart your progress using the following tests:

1 Spine roll (from page 18)

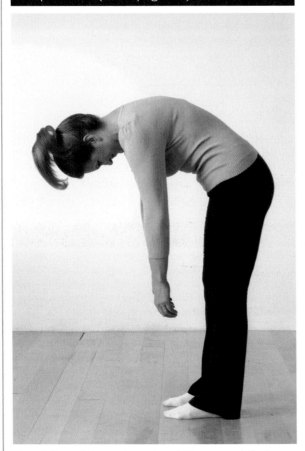

Try a Spine roll-down. Any twinges? Can you curl further than you did before?

2 Cossack Arms (from page 33)

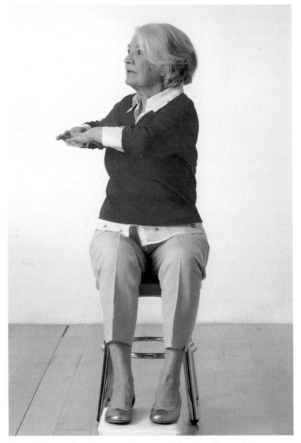

Sit with your back to a mirror and do the Cossack Arms exercise. Can you twist round far enough to see yourself in the mirror? Don't let your hip bones move, and keep your fingertips in line with your breastbone.

One of the main differences that you will have noticed after a month of Pilates is that your "muscle memories" are getting stronger. When an exercise instructs you to "slide your shoulder blades down your back", "engage your abdominals", or "pull up your pelvic floor", you should remember what this feels like and how you can achieve it.

Feel free to mix and match exercises to create your own routines according to your energy level on the day and the areas you need to ease or strengthen. Every main session should include Glute squeezes and Hamstring curls, plus some abdominal and lats exercises, but skip them in shorter or easier workouts. Remember to include some stretches in the opposite direction if you have been working intensively on one area: for example, after a lot of abdominal work, do a back stretch; after intensive leg work, do a hamstring stretch. And forget about that 1980s mantra "No pain, no gain". In Pilates, if you feel any pain at all, you must stop what you're doing!

How are your Ab curls coming along? Can you do them without straining your neck or inner thighs? Can you feel the stomach muscles getting stronger?

3 Ab curls (from page 92)

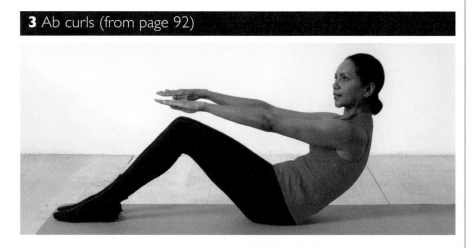

How far back can you pull each leg in the Hamstring stretch? Can you stretch further now than when you started Pilates?

4 Hamstring stretch (from page 98)

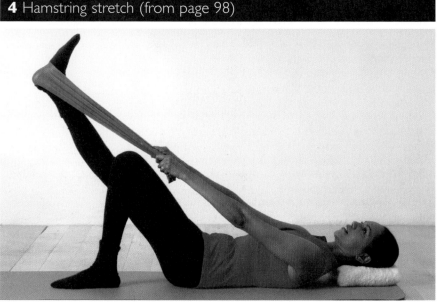

An easy workout

Let yourself off the hook if you're having a tough day. This breathing and stretching routine is performed on the floor and doesn't have any tricky moves, but it will still loosen you up and make you feel more energized.

Do 10 static abs.

1 Static abs (from page 50)

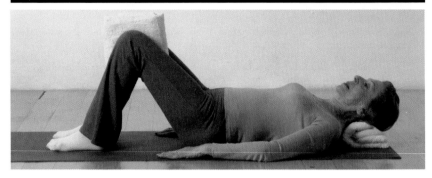

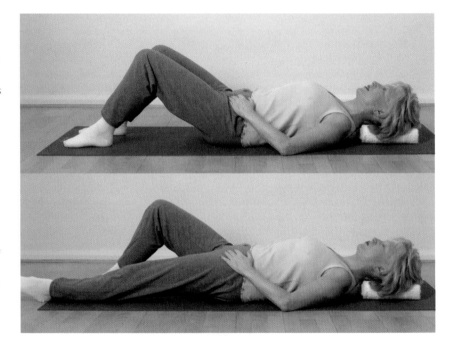

2 Leg slides

1 This works the inner thigh and the hip joint. Lie on your back with your knees bent and your hands on your stomach just below your hip bones. Look up at the ceiling and breathe in.

2 As you breathe out, engage your abdominals and slide your left leg down so that it extends along the floor. Squeeze your left glute as you lower your leg. Breathe in and draw your leg back up to the starting position.

Repeat five times on each leg.

3 Back stretch (from page 26)

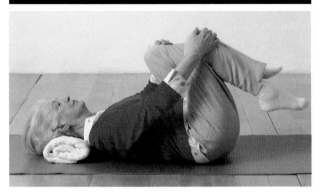

Lie on your back on the floor to do a basic Back stretch with your knees hugged to your chest.

4 Back stretch clock face (from page 27)

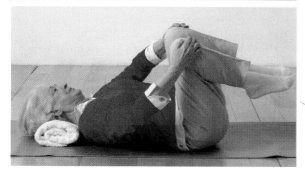

Do another Back stretch, but this time imagine a clock face up above you. Move your knees slowly round each of the figures in a clockwise direction, then back again in an anticlockwise direction.

5 Hip rolls (from page 69)

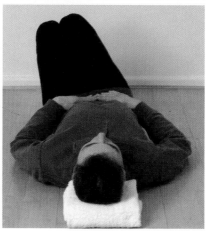

Do 10 Hip rolls in alternating directions.

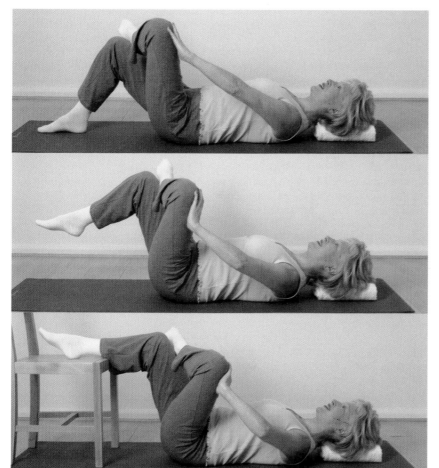

6 Buttock stretch

1 Lie on your back with your knees bent and feet hip-width apart. Place your left ankle across the front of the right thigh. Place your left hand on your left knee and open the knee. Breathe in.

2 As you breathe out, pull your right knee to your chest as you gently push the left knee back with your hand.

Repeat with the other leg.

Variation
If you find it difficult to hold your right leg up as you stretch the buttock, place your right foot on a chair positioned close by.

An easy workout

7 Side-lying static abs (from page 56)

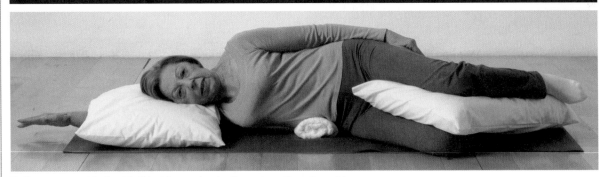

Roll onto your side for 10 Side-lying static abs. Repeat on the other side.

8 The Shell

Now try a new exercise called the Shell, which works your glutes and the backs of your thighs.

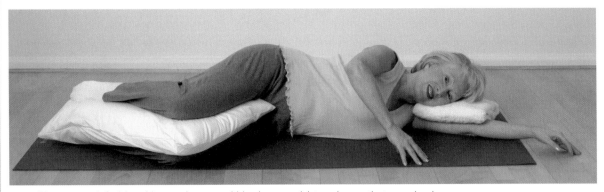

1 Lie on your left side, with your knees and hips bent at right angles so that your heels are level with your tailbone. Place a pillow between your knees and your feet. If necessary, place a small cushion under your waist and another under your head. Place the fingertips of your right hand on the floor in front of you. Breathe in.

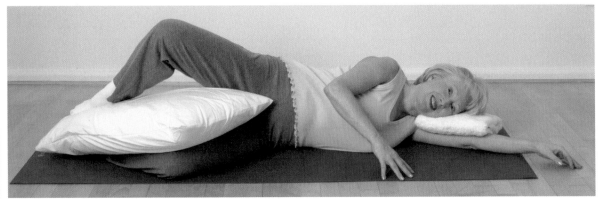

2 As you breathe out, engage your abdominals, gently squeeze your glutes, and use the movement to open your right thigh as far as you can while keeping your hips and feet in the same position. Breathe in to return to the starting position.

Repeat five times on each side.

9 Upper body release (from page 55)

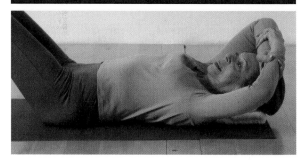

Do 10 repetitions of the Upper body release to each side.

10 Painting the ceiling

1 This loosens the neck. Sit upright on a stool and pull your shoulder blades down your back. Relax your arms and hands at your sides. Lengthen the back of your neck and tilt your head gently to one side.

2 Look briefly down at your knees. Tilt your head in a smooth movement from side to side again.

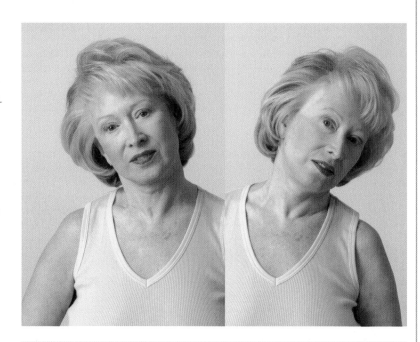

3 Move your head in tiny circular movements.

4 Move your head gently up and down and in circles for as long as it feels comfortable.

CAUTION: The photographs here show the direction of the movements, but keep your movements very small – only a couple of centimetres in each direction. Don't ever try to circle your head around. Don't try this exercise at all if you have neck problems.

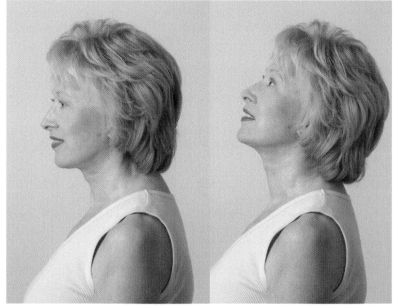

A moderate workout

After you've been doing Pilates for a few weeks and you have developed reasonable abdominal strength, you shouldn't find this routine too challenging. If any exercise causes lower back pain, it could mean that your abdominals aren't strong enough yet, in which case you should leave the workout alone for the time being.

1 Glute squeeze (from page 58)

Start by lying on your stomach and doing 10 Glute squeezes.

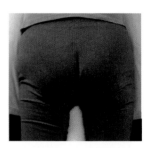

2 Hamstring curls (from page 59)

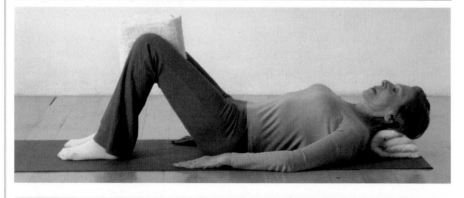

Do 10 Hamstring curls with each leg. Use your pelvic floor muscles as you work.

3 Semi-supine static abs (from page 50)

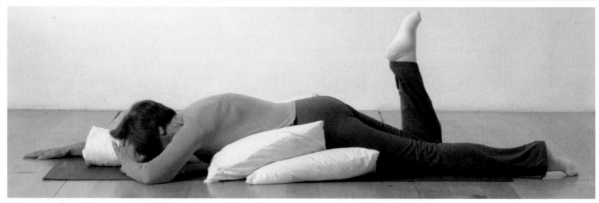

Roll onto your back for 10 repetitions of Semi-supine static abs.

4 Pelvic tilts (from page 51)

Do 10 Pelvic tilts.

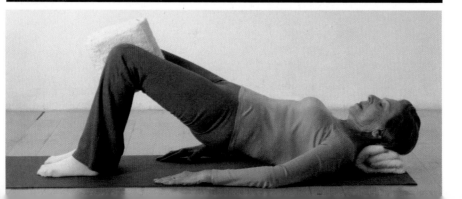

5 Leg lifts

Now it's time to work the abs with a new exercise called Leg lifts:

1 Lie on your back in the semi-supine position, with your hands resting lightly on your abdomen. Breathe in.

2 As you breathe out, engage your abdominals and lift your left leg off the floor. Point your toes, keeping your knee bent at the same angle. Don't tense the right leg and don't let your pelvis move. Feel the muscles in your abdomen creating the movement.

Breathe in to lower your leg again and repeat five times on each side.

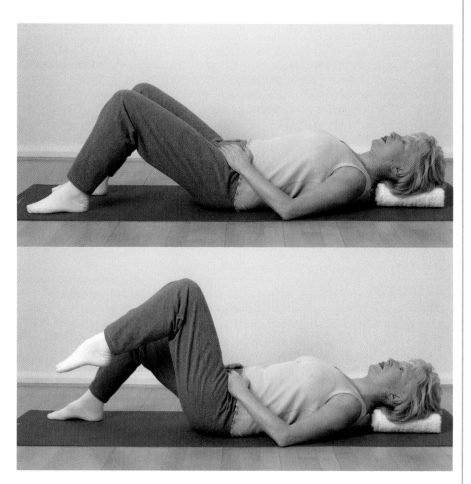

6 Ab curls (from page 90)

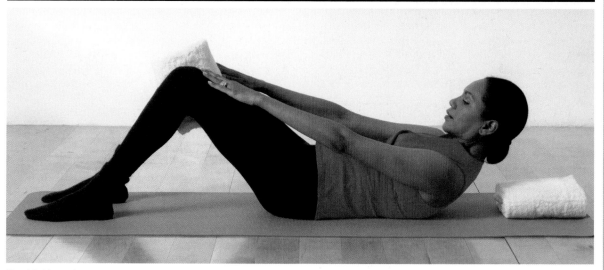

Do 10 Ab curls.

A moderate workout

7 Inner thigh stretch

This movement stretches the inner thigh and helps to
mobilize the hip joint.

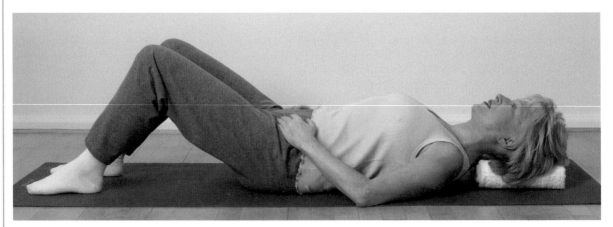

Lie on your back with your knees bent and your hands resting on
your hip bones. Place a folded towel under your head.

8 Sitting lats (from page 63)

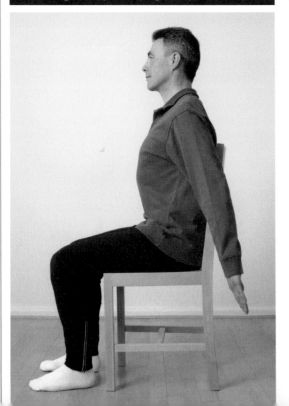

9 Working the upper torso (from page 64)

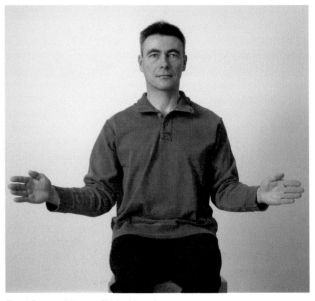

Do 10 repetitions of Working the upper torso.

Sit on a stool or armless chair and do some shoulder
shrugs (see p.62), then 10 repetitions of Sitting lats.

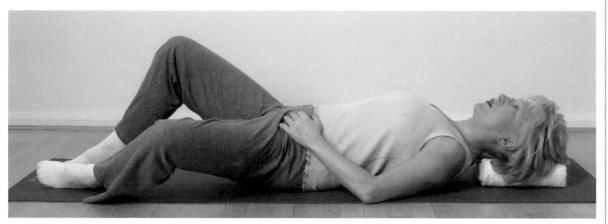

2 As you breathe out, let your left knee drop naturally out to the side,
as far as is comfortable. Don't allow your opposite hip to move.
Breathe in as you raise your knee back to the start position.
Repeat 10 times on each side.

10 Cossack Arms (from page 66)

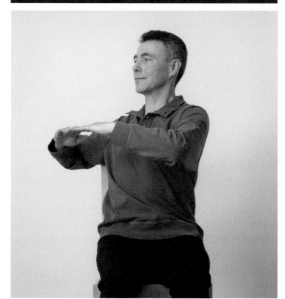

Do 10 repetitions of Cossack Arms.

11 Side bends (from page 67)

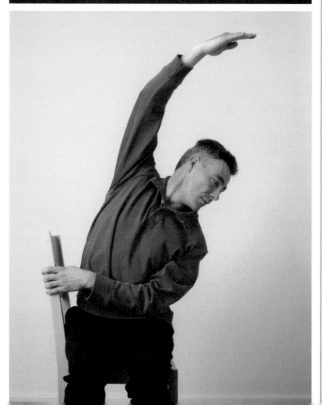

Do five Side bends to each side.

A challenging workout

This is a workout for the abdomen and the back to strengthen the core muscles that hold your spine and pelvis in place. Don't try it until you've been doing Pilates for a couple of months and can manage 10 Ab curls without straining.

1 Glute squeeze
(from page 58)

Begin with 10 Glute squeezes.

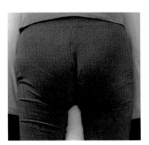

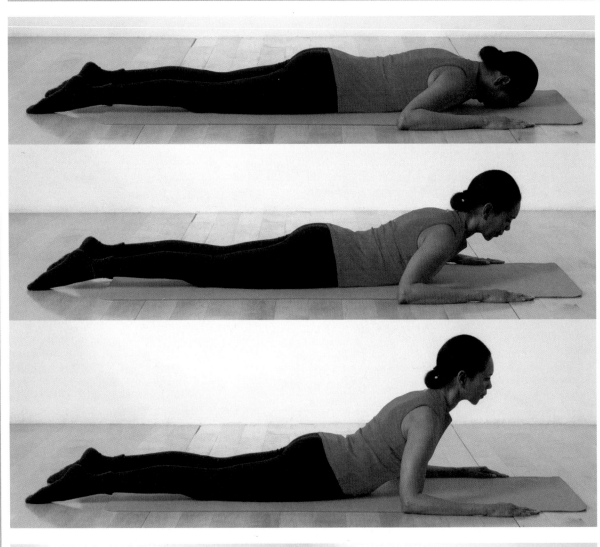

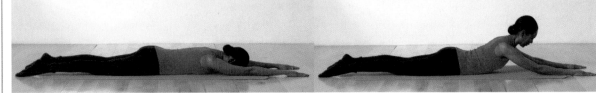

2 Hamstring curls (from page 59)

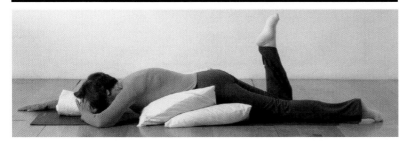

Next do 10
Hamstring curls.

3 Cobra

Stretch out the abs with this stretch
known as the Cobra:

1 Lie face down with your
forehead resting on the floor
and your arms bent by the sides
of your head, palms facing downward.
Breathe in.

2 As you breathe out, squeeze
your glutes slightly and lift your
upper body off the floor
without moving your arms.

3 Lift higher, keeping your elbows
on the floor and pulling your
shoulder blades down. Breathe
in to return to the starting position.

Repeat 10 times.

Variation
Keep your forehead on the floor and
your arms extended out in front of
you on the floor. Keep your arms
straight as you lift the upper body.
Press your palms down. To work the
sides of the back, turn your palms on
their sides and repeat.

4 Rest position

To finish the workout, end with a last back stretch
in Rest position:

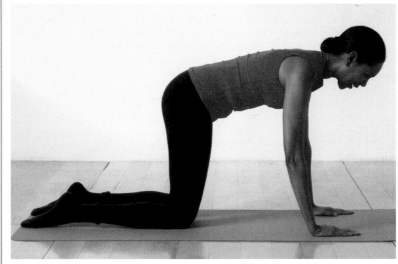

1 Push down into your hands and forearms to raise yourself up so that you are
kneeling on all fours. Don't drop your head.

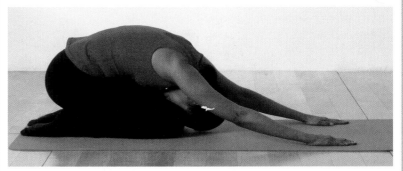

2 Leaving your hands in the same position, lower your bottom backward
onto your heels. Lower your upper body until your forehead is resting on
the floor and stretch your hands in front of you as far as you can. Rest for
a couple of minutes.

A challenging workout

5 Pelvic tilt

This version of the Pelvic tilt takes you higher off the floor than the one you tried earlier, and it uses the arms as well:

1 Lie on your back in the semi-supine position, with a folded towel between your knees and another under your head. Relax your arms by your sides. Breathe in.

2 As you breathe out, engage your abdominals, pull up your pelvic floor and start curling your tailbone upward between your legs. Keep curling right up until you are resting on your shoulder blades, and your shoulders and knees are in a straight line.

3 Breathe in and lift your arms up toward the ceiling.

4 Breathe out and slowly curl your body back down to the floor, leaving your arms still stretching up toward the ceiling.

Breathe in to bring your arms back to your sides, or you can stretch your arms back behind you onto the floor and circle them round to your sides. Repeat 10 times.

CAUTION: This version of the pelvic tilt should not be attempted by anyone with neck or shoulder problems.

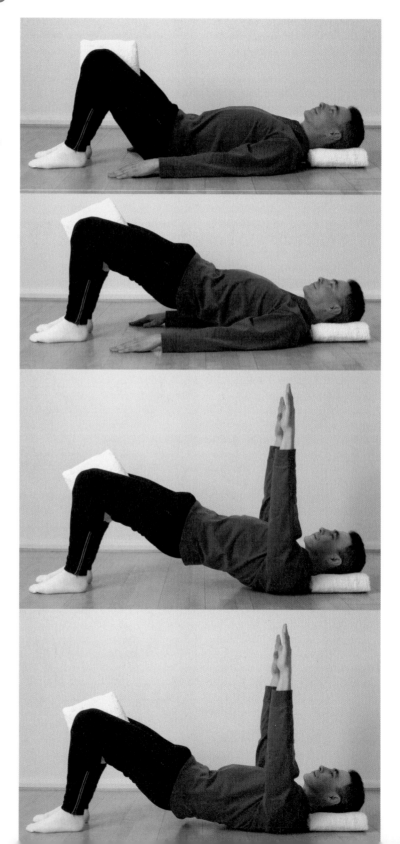

6 Ab curls (from page 90)

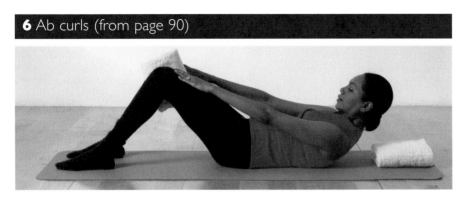

Do 10 Ab curls. Rest your hands on your hips and, as you breathe out and start to curl upward, walk your fingers up your thighs towards your knees.

7 Cross-fibre ab curls (from page 91)

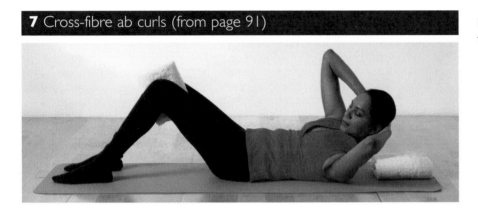

Do 5 Cross-fibre Ab curls to each side.

8 Hip roll

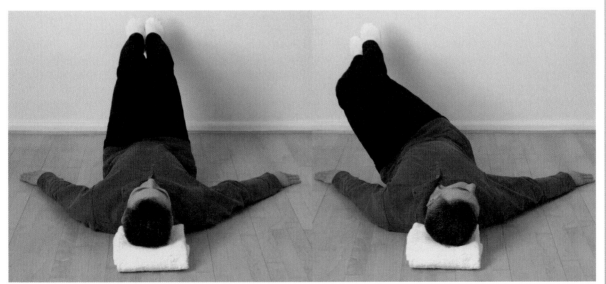

1 Lie in a semi-supine position on the floor with your arms at your sides and your knees bent. Lift one knee and then the other so that both feet are in the air.

2 Breathe out, engage your abdominals, and drop your knees to the left. Turn your head slightly to the right. Repeat three times on each side.

A challenging workout

9 Single leg stretches

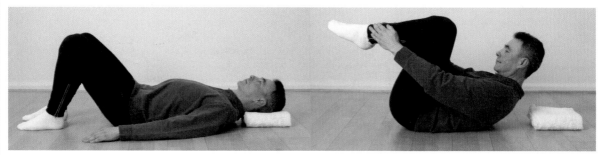

Try a new exercise called Single leg stretches:

| Lie on your back in a semi-supine position with a folded towel under your head.

2 Lift first one knee then the other to your chest and hold your knees with your hands. Slide your hands down to your ankles. Breathe in. As you breathe out, engage your abdominals and curl your upper body off the floor. Breathe in, but keep your abdominals engaged.

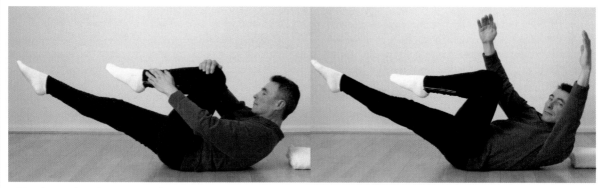

3 As you breathe out, stretch out your right leg and transfer your right hand to your left knee. Breathe in and change legs, straightening your left leg and transferring your hands to your right knee and right ankle.

Do 10 repetitions on each side, keeping your abdominals engaged throughout.

Variation
Lift both hands up and bend and straighten each leg alternately so that you create a cycling motion.

11 Inner thigh – lying (from page 97)

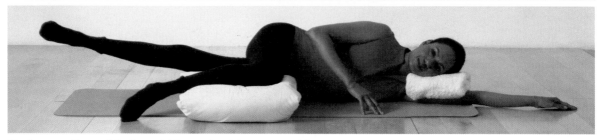

Do five repetitions of the Inner thigh exercises lying on your side.

10 Hamstring stretch

Try a Hamstring stretch:

1 Lie on your back in a semi-supine position. Raise the left knee to your chest and clasp both hands behind it. Breathe in.

2 As you breathe out, engage your abdominals and straighten the left leg up to vertical, then see if you can pull it toward your chest a bit.

3 Flex and point the foot four to eight times. Lower the left leg, then repeat with the right leg.

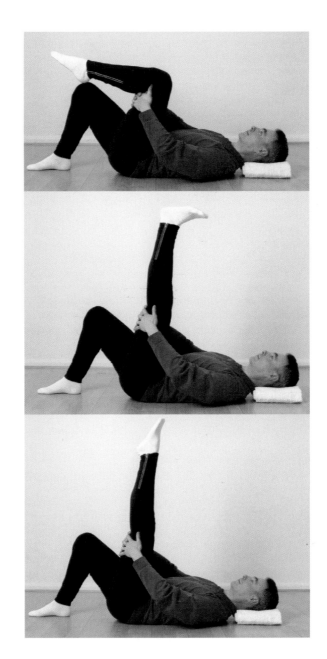

12 Double leg lift (from page 93)

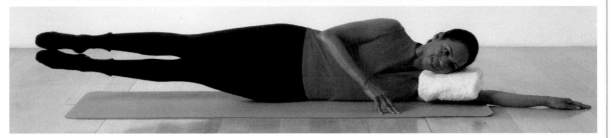

Do five Double leg lifts on each side.

A Challenging Workout

13 Side leg kicks

For this exercise, you'll need to have strong abdominals to control your movements.

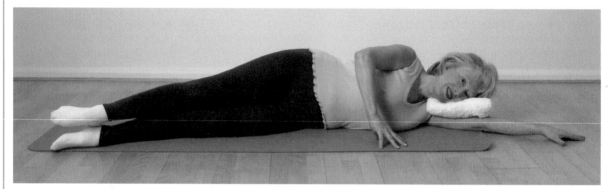

1 Lie on your left side, with your legs together. Extend your left arm along the floor and place a folded towel between your arm and your head. Breathe in.

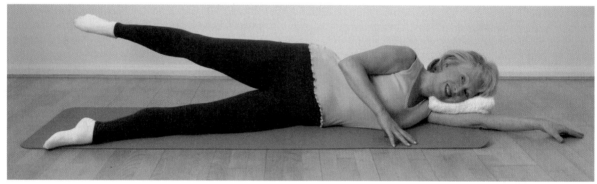

2 As you breathe out, engage your abdominals, lift your right leg up, and stretch it backward as far as you can without straining. Breathe in.

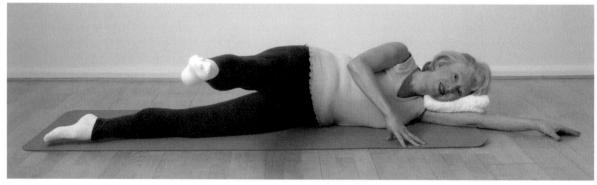

3 Breathe in and bring the leg forward as far as you can.

Repeat five times, then turn onto your right side and repeat with the left leg.

14 The Star

Now try a new exercise called the Star, which is like a strange kind of swimming:

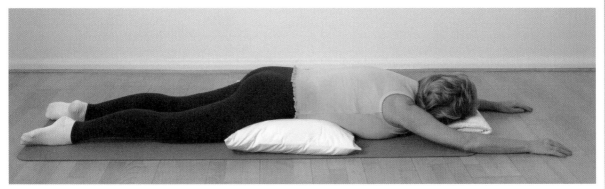

Lie on your front. Place a pillow under your abdomen and a folded towel or a book under your forehead. Extend your arms in front of you with your hands roughly shoulder-width apart and your palms resting on the floor. Your legs should be extended and your feet hip-width apart. Breathe in.

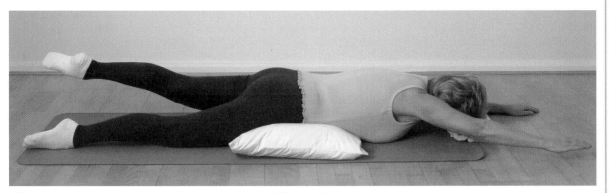

2 As you breathe out, engage your abdominals, and lift your right arm and left leg off the floor. Try to raise them by the same distance – it doesn't have to be far.

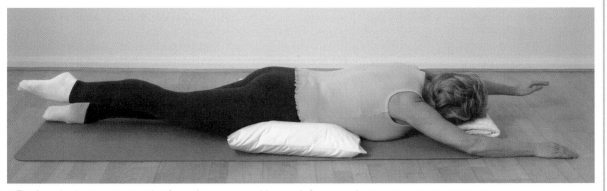

3 Breathe in to return to the floor, then repeat with your left arm and right leg. Do 10 repetitions on each side.

A challenging workout

15 Shoulder release

Another new exercise called the Shoulder release will do exactly what its name suggests:

1 Lie on your left side with your knees and hips bent and a folded towel under your head. Extend your arms in front of you with your palms together. Breathe in.

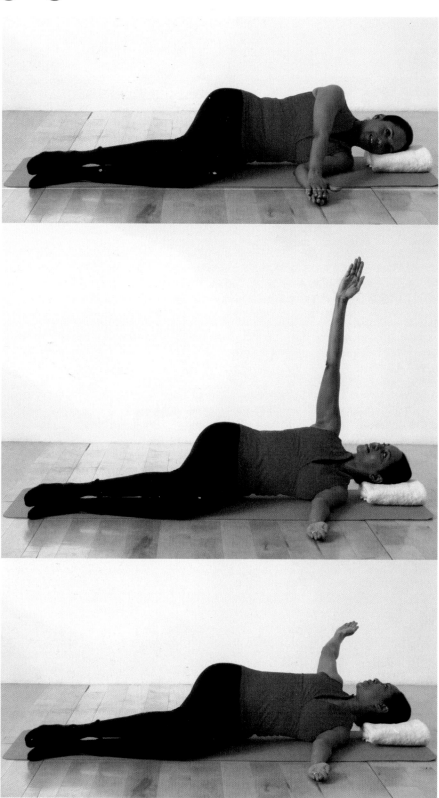

2 As you breathe out, engage your abdominals and lift your right arm up toward the ceiling. Follow the movement of your arm with your head, but don't move your hips and feet.

3 Move your hand over your upper body toward the floor behind you. Keep your abs engaged. Breathe in to return to the start position.

Repeat five times on each side.

16 The Cat

Come back onto all fours to try an exercise called the Cat:

CAUTION: Don't scoop your back downward if you have lordosis. Place a rolled-up towel under your hands if you have wrist problems, and if it still hurts, give this exercise – and the next one – a miss for now.

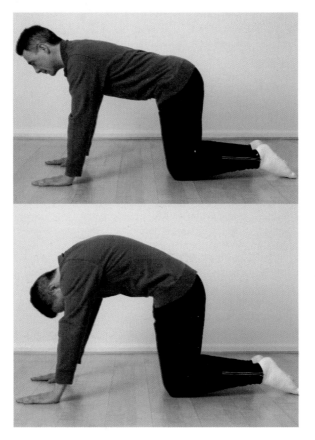

1 Kneel on all fours with your hands slightly in front of your shoulders, and with shoulders, knees, and hips roughly in line. Keep your neck straight.

2 Breathe in and curve your spine upward, starting the movement with your pelvis, then your stomach, and upper back. Drop your head. Don't lean forward.

Breathe out, engage your abdominals and lower your back down into a natural curved shape – not too arched – so that your head and bottom lift upward. Breathe in to return to the start position.

Repeat 10 times.

17 The Dog

The Dog needs more abdominal strength than the Cat. Give it a try, but if you don't feel comfortable or balanced, leave it for a few weeks then try again.

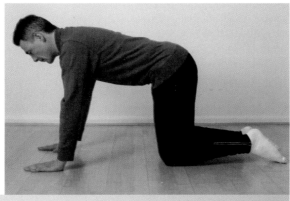

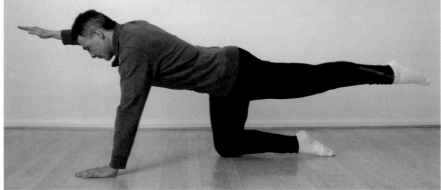

1 Kneel on all fours with your back in a natural curve and your neck straight. Breathe in.

2 As you breathe out, engage your abdominals and extend your right arm and your left leg. Try to hold them level at shoulder and hip height without losing your balance or letting your back arch. Breathe in to return to the start position.

Repeat five times on each side.

129

A challenging workout

18 Threading the needle

This exercise gives a stretch across the shoulders and the thoracic muscles.

1 Start on all fours in the Cat position. Make sure that your knees are positioned hip-width apart. Lift your right hand off the floor slightly and keep your elbow soft. Breathe in.

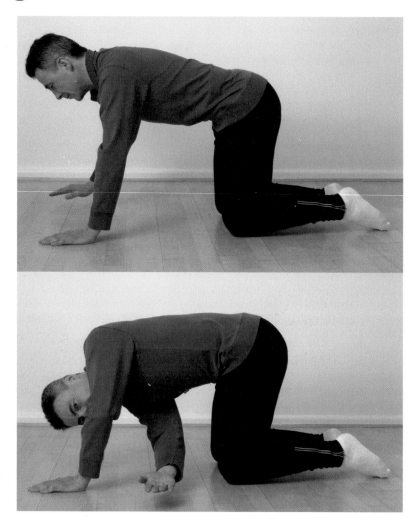

2 As you breathe out, engage your abdominals, turn the palm of your hand upward, and push your hand through the space created between your left arm and left leg. Extend your fingers as you push through and allow your head to follow the movement of your hand. Breathe in and return to the starting position.

Repeat three times on each side.

20 Cobra (from page 120)

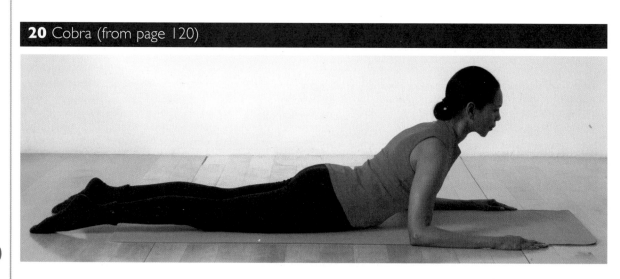

19 Hip roll on physio ball

Feel this stretch through the length of your spine.
Ask someone to hold the chair seat firmly as you
do this exercise.

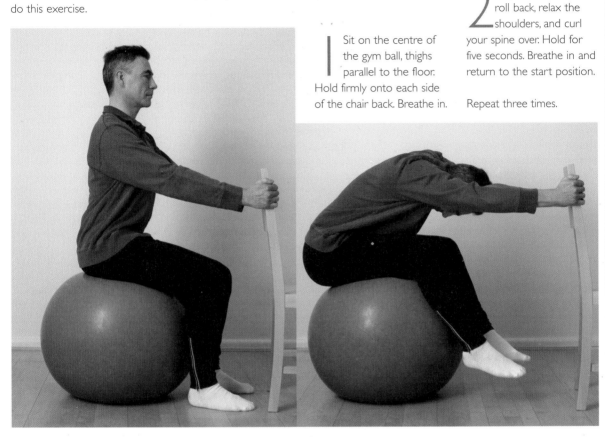

1 Sit on the centre of the gym ball, thighs parallel to the floor. Hold firmly onto each side of the chair back. Breathe in.

2 As you breathe out, roll back, relax the shoulders, and curl your spine over. Hold for five seconds. Breathe in and return to the start position.

Repeat three times.

21 Rest position (from page 121)

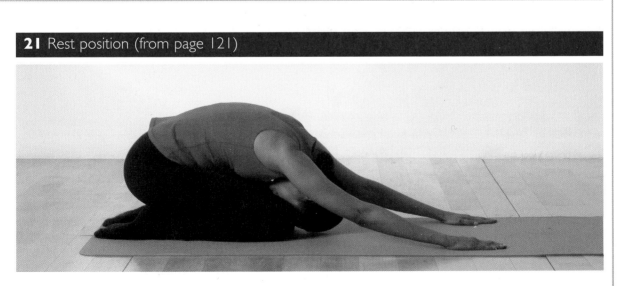

131

Case histories

"I was in my seventies, and suffering with osteoporosis and severely arthritic hips when a friend recommended that I try learning Pilates. I had done yoga for many years but had to give it up as my pain and immobility increased. I arrived at Alan's studio hobbling on a walking stick, not sure what to expect, but I was immediately impressed by the skill of the instructors and the personal attention I received. Gradually, I built up the muscle strength to cope with two hip replacement operations. After each one, there were about six weeks when I had to walk on crutches but I resumed Pilates in my weak and wobbly state. Week by week my strength returned and my muscles got stronger and I could do more for longer at the studio. Now, three years on, I have achieved the accomplishment of walking along the balance bar unaided. I am stronger and have more mobility than I ever thought possible, and retaining it has become my priority as I move into old age." **Valerie**

"I am a dentist, and dentistry is very bad for your back. You have to sit very still to get fine control of your fingers, just as you would when threading a needle, so your muscles are tensed throughout the working day. You also tend to turn to one side as you work. After a while your posture is affected and a lot of dentists end up with permanently hunched shoulders and shortened necks. I always used to be in pain at the end of the day, but since I started doing Pilates four or five years ago, I sit with better posture and have much less tension in my muscles. I've really noticed how much straighter my posture is and I think I'm actually taller. The staff in Alan's studio keep a close eye on me to correct any one-sidedness and make sure my muscles are balanced. Just one Pilates session a week is enough to keep me straight, toned and pain-free." **Gerard**

"In August 2002, aged 79, I fell and broke my leg in four places, and all in a zig-zag fashion. After the operation, I was in terrible pain and couldn't imagine I would ever walk again. I rang Alan Herdman to tell him I wouldn't be coming to the studio and explained what had happened. He said, 'Come here at once, and bring your x-rays.' Alan seemed certain that I would walk again, but I didn't believe him. He worked out a programme that I would do with one of his teachers, Jenny, and I got to work. At the end of October when I went back to the hospital for an x-ray, the surgeon was amazed to see that my bones were beginning to fuse. By the end of

November, I could walk, albeit with a limp, but Alan told me I didn't need to limp, it was all in my mind. The surgeon couldn't believe the progress I had made and asked a lot of questions about the exercises I had been doing. Now I walk without a limp and go to the gym every single day. To be honest, I couldn't have coped with life in a wheelchair, so Alan and his assistants literally gave me my life back." **Janine**

"I've had an ongoing back problem for as long as I can remember, and my osteopath suggested I went to Alan's studio. Part of the problem is that I play the viola and have to hold this huge instrument under my chin, which is idiotic for someone with back problems. Pilates helped me to build up my muscles – otherwise, I simply couldn't have continued with the viola." **Hilly**

"I work in publishing, so there's lots of computer work and leaning over the desk to read page proofs, and as a result I've had neck problems since my early 30s. By the time I discovered Pilates, I had been trekking to osteopaths and physiotherapists for almost 10 years, seeking a cure for recurrent trapped nerves down my arms. My shoulders were bunched up tight, two of the vertebrae in my neck were degenerating, and I was fed up with the constant nausea, dizziness, and pins and needles in my hands and arms caused by the trapped nerves. The osteopaths cracked the joints, providing short-term relief, and physiotherapists tried a variety of techniques, many of them painful. One physiotherapist applied strong sticky tape to my back to try and pull the shoulder blades down – but it wasn't until I started working with Alan Herdman that anyone taught me to strengthen the muscles in my mid back to enable me to hold my shoulders down myself. I didn't think I had any lats when I first tried Pilates, but Alan said 'Don't worry, they're in there!' Now I am largely pain-free, but if I ever get a twinge after a long day at work, I know how to exercise to ease it out by myself without relying on anyone else." **Gill**

"I was a couch potato, definitely not an exercise fan, and I had seriously arthritic knees. The physio I saw after my first knee replacement recommended that I consult Alan Herdman. At first, I'm sure he disguised his shock at how unfit I was. He helped me to prepare for my second knee replacement and then to strengthen my knees after surgery, but the effects were much more dramatic than that. My whole body shape

133

Case histories

has changed, my back is much stronger, my knees are more or less painfree, and now I've become passionate about exercise. It doesn't matter how frazzled you feel when you arrive at Alan's studio, you always feel energized and ready for the day ahead by the time you leave. Alan helped me to prepare when I was appearing in a musical that involved six hours of non-stop rehearsing every day, and I would never have managed it without the strength I had built up. Basically, he revolutionized my life." **Felicity**

"I had a skiing accident and slipped a disc when I was thirty years old. For the next ten years, I had regular treatments with a back specialist who gave me injections between the vertebrae to prop up my back, but one day it suddenly went again while I was driving. I was in agony and a friend recommended a cranial osteopath, so I tried that for the next four years. At the same time, I was doing yoga, but the osteopath told me that wasn't quite the right thing for me – it was making me more flexible, but I didn't have enough strength in the muscles that support the spine – so she referred me to Alan Herdman. That was seven years ago. When I first arrived at his studio, I could hardly move. I'd been off work for almost a year, and I had to get a cab there and back because my whole body had seized up from the amount of time I'd been forced to spend lying down. Alan started me off with some very small movements, and gradually my core strength grew. I've got amazing strength now, seven years on, after two sessions of Pilates every week. I go to the studio even when my back's hurting because I have the confidence to judge what I can and can't do. Alan has also helped me to manage my job safely. I'm a costume designer, so there's a lot of standing working at tables, and he taught me how to position my cutting table at the right height. I can manage fittings now, with all the bending, kneeling and climbing around, and Alan has also shown me correct sitting positions. If it hadn't been for him, I'd have given up and changed my profession. He's the man!" **Claire C**

"In my fifties I got frozen shoulder very badly and then, just as I was recovering, my knee cartilage needed surgery. During the operation, my arm got broken and it couldn't be set, so it took a long time to heal. Both my right knee and my left arm were so weak that the consultant told me I would always be severely disabled. I needed carers to dress me and help me get up and downstairs. Six months later I met someone who recommended that I should go to see Alan Herdman at his Pilates studio, so I called him up and asked 'Would you like a difficult case?' When he started working with me, I couldn't lift my arm at all and had very restricted movement in it. Alan designed a gentle, very sensitive programme for me and four years later, I now have almost full use of the arm. My first goal was to be able to hold my grandchild, and I achieved it. I've taken up golf again and gone back to sailing. Little things like being able to wash my own hair again and put on underarm deodorant have been important milestones. My leg is now straight and gradually, centimetre by centimetre, I'm increasing the movement in my arm every day. It's just incredible what Pilates does!" **Clare W**

"A year and a half ago, I tripped and fell, causing a serious fracture of my right arm. It was badly set at first, then had to be realigned a few weeks later. They did a bone density test in the hospital and discovered I have osteopenia, a precursor of osteoporosis, which came as a great shock to me because I was only 52 and, like most people, I'd always assumed it was a disease of post-menopausal women. Anyway, it turns out men get it as well. I couldn't use my arm at all while it was in a brace, so I needed help with almost everything. I couldn't get dressed, take a shower on my own, or go to bed at night without help. Alan devised a set of exercises for me to strengthen the shoulder muscles, the lats, and the arm itself, and in less than five months I had 100% movement back. The specialist couldn't believe his eyes as he watched me rotating my arm, lifting it out sideways, and even sliding my thumb up my back. The great thing about Pilates is that it makes you very aware of your body, so you adopt the correct positions for lifting, pulling, pushing, sitting, and standing. It can't cure my osteopenia, but by strengthening the muscles that support the bones, it should help me to avoid any more fractures in future." **Andrew**

"I was smashed to pieces in a car crash in 1988. I broke my foot, hip, pelvis, and left arm, I needed a plate inserted in my left leg, and I also had whiplash. It took me two years before I could hobble back to work on sticks. A couple of years later, my physiotherapist recommended Pilates and I came to Alan's studio for the first time, and it was my lifesaver. To let you know how far I've come, five years ago I climbed the Annapurna Range, albeit with guides carrying my rucksack (I still can't carry anything because of lower back trouble). This year I've had a remarkably successful hip operation; within six weeks, I was walking without sticks or crutches. I highly recommend anyone who has hip surgery to do Pilates first to strengthen the muscles and speed their recovery time." **Pamela**

Glossary

Abduction
A movement away from the centre line of the body. In Sitting deltoids (see p.80), you abduct your arms away from the body, and in Outer thigh lifts (see p.57), you abduct your leg. The muscles used are known as abductors.

Adduction
A movement towards the centre line of the body. In Adductor squeeze (see p.54) you adduct your arm, and in Inner thighs – sitting (see p.68), you adduct your legs. The muscles used are known as adductors.

Aerobic exercise
Exercise that raises the heart rate and makes you breathe harder to deliver more oxygen to the muscles. Running, cycling and swimming are all aerobic if you work hard enough.

Balance bar
A narrow beam to practice walking along while keeping your balance.

Core stability
By strengthening the muscles in the centre of the body, you can keep the pelvis and spine in correct alignment and protect yourself from injury. Core stability is one of the key goals in Pilates.

Deltoids
Muscles across the shoulders that move the arms up and down and out to the sides. These muscles are used in Sitting deltoids (see p.80).

Engaging the abdominals
Pulling the stomach muscles toward the back. This instruction is often given at the beginning of a Pilates exercise.

Extension
If you are asked to extend an arm or a leg in an exercise, it means you should straighten it (but you will usually be told not to "lock" it – see below).

Flexion
Flexion generally means bending. If you are asked to flex your foot, you should bend it back towards your shin.

Glutes
The gluteus maximus muscles across the bottom help to straighten the hip and rotate the hip joint outwards. These are used in many Pilates exercises, as well as in many movements in everyday life, and Glute squeezes (see p.24) will help to strengthen them.

Hamstrings
Muscles down the backs of the thighs that help to bend the knee and straighten the hip. It's important to keep them strong or you risk knee injuries. Hamstring curls (see p.59) will strengthen them.

Isometric
A movement that contracts the muscle without shortening it.

Kyphosis
Pronounced forward curve of the upper back (see p.15, p.82).

Latissimus dorsi (lats)
Muscles of the mid back that hold the shoulder blades down, pull the arms backward and rotate them inward. Sitting lats (see p.63) are one of the key exercises to master for strengthening these.

Ligament
A tough fibrous band inside a joint that holds the bones together and stops joints from moving too far. Ligament injuries can be very debilitating.

Lock
In Pilates, you are taught never to lock knee and elbow joints. This means that they should never be totally straightened, but kept slightly "soft".

Lordosis
Pronounced curvature of the lower back, causing the stomach and bottom to stick out (see p.15, p.89).

Muscle memory
As you learn the correct way to do an exercise, you create a "memory" of the muscles you need to use, how you activate them and what the movements feel like, to allow you to do the same move easily next time.

Obliques
Muscles round the sides of the waist that help to turn the body to the sides. You'll use these in Cross-fibre ab curls (see p.91).

Pelvic alignment
The pelvis can tilt backward and forward (as in Pelvic tilts, p.51), but for daily movements and activities, it should be held by the surrounding muscles in an alignment that doesn't put any strain on the spine. You may not have correct pelvic alignment if you wear high heels a lot, frequently sit with your legs crossed, or if you have poor posture.

Pelvic floor
The hammock of muscles between the legs. Keeping these muscles strong can prevent incontinence and sexual dysfunction in later life.

Physio ball
A large rubber ball that can be used to elevate the feet in several Pilates exercises.

Powerhouse muscles
Three sets of abdominal muscles, plus the glutes, hamstrings and pelvic floors together form the powerhouse muscles that give you core stability.

Prone
Lying face down on the floor.

Quadriceps (quads)
Muscles at the fronts of the thighs that straighten the knee. They are used for walking, running, cycling, standing up from a chair and many other day-to-day activities.

Rectus abdominus
A muscle running from the breastbone down to the pubic bone that is used to bend the body forward.

Reformer
A machine in the Pilates studio that uses springs and weights to provide resistance while helping you to exercise safely.

Rotation
Turning around a central axis, such as rotating the upper body around the spine, as in Cossack Arms (see p.33).

Scoliosis
Sideways curvature of the spine (see p.88, p.93).

Semi-supine
Lying on your back with your knees bent and feet on the floor. This is a common starting position for Pilates exercises.

Serratus anterior
Muscles in the sides of the torso that pull the shoulder blades forward. The Pillow squeeze (see p.84) strengthens these muscles.

Soft
A soft joint should not be totally straightened or "locked". If you are asked to make your neck or your foot soft, make sure they are relaxed, and without tension or straining.

Static abs
Pulling your stomach toward your back. This can be done throughout the day, while you are lying on your back or on your side, sitting, standing up, or kneeling on all fours. The more you do Static ab exercises, the easier you will find it to control your abdominal muscles, and the stronger they will become.

Supine
Lying on your back with your legs straight.

Thoracic
Thorax is the medical name for the chest, so thoracic muscles are in the chest area.

Transverse abdominals
These muscles hold your internal organs in place and are used in Pilates to pull your stomach toward your back.

Trapezius
A large diamond-shaped muscle across the upper back for raising the shoulders, rotating the shoulder blades, and lifting your arms above your head.

Index

Index

Acknowledgments

Alan Herdman would like to thank all the models for their dedication and hard work: Annie Walsh, Gilles Crawford, Hazel Collins, Janine Ingram, Margaret Brierley, Marjorie Baker and Jane Paterson.

Picture credits

Corbis U.K. Ltd. 44, 45 left, 45 right.
Octopus Publishing Group Limited/David Jordan 46 centre, 47 top, 47 bottom; /William Reavell 47 centre; /Simon Smith 46 top; /Adrian Swift 46 bottom.

"The person comes first, the technique second."

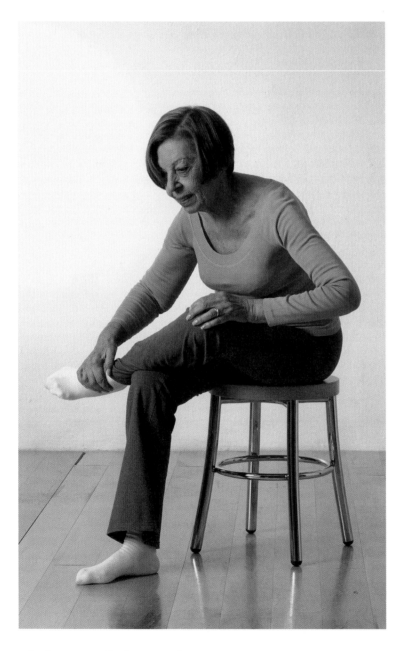

Alan Herdman

"Not mind or body, but mind and body."

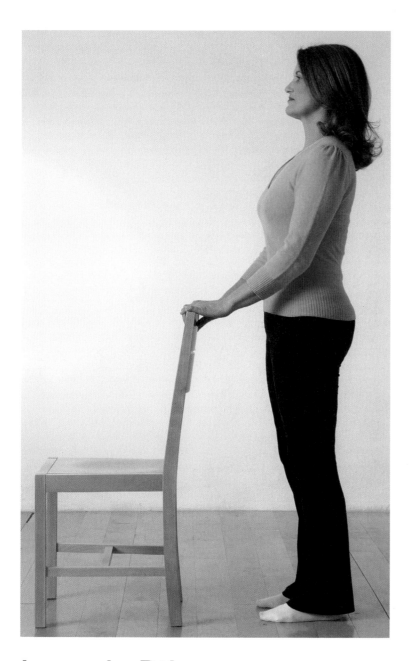

Joseph Pilates